Ancient Einkorn

TODAY'S STAFF OF LIFE

Hybrid Grains, GMOs, and Chemicals
TRUTH OR CONSEQUENCES

D. GARY YOUNG

ISBN #978-0-9905100-0-0

Printed in the United States of America

Young Living Essential Oils
Thanksgiving Point Business Park
3125 Executive Parkway
Lehi, UT 84043

Cover: Gary found this einkorn in Lerik, Azerbaijan, in 2001.

TABLE OF CONTENTS

Acknowledgments 1

Preface 3

Introduction 5

1. My Quest to Find Einkorn 15

2. The Decline of Nutrition 39

3. Modern Hybrid Wheat 49

4. Gluten: Friend or Foe 55

5. Enzymes 77

6. Diseases and Disorders Triggered by Hybrid Gluten 88

7. The Silent Killers the Pharmaceutical Companies Love 117

8. The Road to Recovery and a Healthy Life 155

ACKNOWLEDGMENTS

This journey of discovery has taken me to many remote and unusual places in the world, and the people who have helped and supported me are not only colleagues but are also great friends.

Jean-Noël Landel and his wife Jane have been integral to my success in the European essential oil community. Jean-Noël made pathways for me into what I considered to be a closed society of oil producers. He openly shared what he knew with me about growers and vendors and introduced me to those who became great mentors, who taught me about growing, harvesting, and distilling. We have worked as partners for almost 25 years, which has led to Young Living owning its own lavender farm in the heart of Provence, France. His honesty, integrity, and friendship are close to my heart.

Jean-Noël, my partner and manager of our farm in France, and his son Nicolas, on whom I massaged lavender oil as a baby, have been very instrumental in our einkorn project and have handled all of the details in France, making it possible for us to offer einkorn products this year, 2014. I feel great gratitude to Jean-Noël and his family for all they have done to make our many projects successful.

Benoît Cassan, president of the French Lavender Growers Association and president of the largest research center on lavender farming in the world, has been a great support in achieving our needs in France. He is owner of one of the two farms that are partners with Young Living and is involved in identifying other partner farms for growing aromatic plants to be distilled for essential oils.

Jean-Marie Blanc, also owner of one of the two farms that are partners with Young Living, has been faithful in taking care of our lavender fields and seeing that the einkorn is harvested, ground into flour, and made ready for shipping to the U.S. Jean-Marie is helping to establish other partner farms as well.

Together with Jean-Noël, Benoît, and Jean-Marie, we have established a partnership as well as a trusted friendship that is very successful, from which tens of thousands of people will benefit.

Karen Boren is the Research Writing Manager for Young Living. She is dedicated to making sure the information written is as accurate as possible. Her work is critical to making sure details of the dates, places, and events are correct. She is passionate about historical research and discovering the unknown, especially in the ancient world of the Middle East, which is exactly what I need. She has done an amazing job researching material for this book. Sometimes the hours are long, but for Karen, getting the job done is the most important.

Alene Frandsen is the chief editor and vice president of Publications and Document Review for Young Living and the "go-to" person to make sure everything is right. Alene has the final say on what goes to print; and when there is a deadline, she burns the "midnight oil," which she did many times to meet the print deadline for this book. She always has a smile on her face and is there to help anyone who asks. She is a great asset to Young Living and a great friend who has helped me immensely.

Marc Schreuder, vice president of science at Young Living, has traveled the world with Gary; his experience and knowledge have been invaluable over the years. He has dedicated many hours to edit this book for its scientific and technical data. His contribution has added much and I greatly appreciate him.

David Petty's beautiful renditions and enhancements to several pictures add a special touch to this book. He works to please and is always willing, no matter how tedious the requests. He has been a dedicated artist for many years at Young Living, and I appreciate him very much for all that he has done to make this book a success.

Paul Springer, our designer and graphic artist, has been a friend for many years and has done a magnificent job, as usual, in making this a very professional and beautiful publication. We appreciate him immensely working to the last minute to take care of every little detail.

My wife, Mary, is the glue that holds everything together. She is unrelenting in her desire to make whatever she is doing the best. She has spent long hours working with Alene and Karen to bring this book to publication. Many people ask me how Mary looks after our two boys with school and all their activities, takes care of the house, works in the office, and helps me with my demanding schedule. I love and appreciate her and the sacrifices she makes for our family and the success of Young Living.

PREFACE

"Look deep into nature, and then you will understand everything better."

Albert Einstein

When I was in the mountains with my father, he would always say, "Listen to the sound of the wind or the call of a wild animal. Look at the tracks; what animal is it and where is it going? Watch the trees and see how they move. Look at the shape of the seed or the plant that grows from it. Nature will always tell you what's real—she'll always tell you the truth."

My father was a man of nature. He understood the mountains. He understood the soil and he understood the plants that grew from that soil. He taught me to watch the seedlings grow and see what happened when they were nourished and taken care of in contrast to things that people did that impeded their growth—things that didn't work.

He didn't like chemicals and saw their destructive influence, even though others touted their value. "Don't believe what you hear, believe what you see. Listen, learn, and understand."

As I watched my mother suffer with no understanding, I started asking questions. When my body was so drugged from my accident and I wondered who I was, I turned back to nature; to look deep into my trauma; to understand and choose a new path.

That new path expanded my mind and gave me a greater depth of understanding that has kept me looking deeper into the gifts of Mother Nature and her healing power and has given me the ability to discern truth. When we alter the truth, when we change Mother Nature—our food—our water—she comes back with a vengeance; and the consequences can be devastating.

Truth is my passion and the research and discovery explained in this book have given me more direction and certainty of the choices I make, for which I will be forever grateful.

— D. Gary Young

While conducting research in Morocco in June of 2014, Gary discovers wheat that looks like the wheat his family grew on the farm in Challis, Idaho, when he was a boy. He enjoyed the bread made from this wheat and had no bloating or intolerant reaction like he would have had with regular wheat products that he used to eat.

INTRODUCTION

I grew up in the mountains near Challis, Idaho, in a four-room log cabin with my parents and five siblings. The first cabin I lived in until the age of four was 16 x 20 feet with a board floor and dirt roof. Dad built the second cabin we lived in that was 30 x 30 feet. However, neither cabin had electricity or running water. We lived off the land, taking only what we needed. My father allowed us to shoot wild game only when we needed the meat for our livelihood.

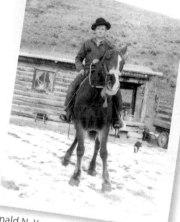

Donald N. Young, Gary's father, in front of their first cabin with the dirt roof.

I had little exposure to food outside of what Mother Nature provided and my mother's kitchen. Planting, growing, harvesting, grinding, shooting, cleaning, drying, canning, and storing was my education. My father always said, "If we don't grow it or shoot it, we don't eat it! Life in the mountains was harsh, and my father seemed harsh; but as a child, I couldn't imagine what it was like for him to provide for six children and a wife who was sick all of the time.

We worked hard to survive, to make a living, and to have enough to eat. But I loved it. I did not know there was any other way. I loved hard work and I loved seeing the accomplishment of hard work, and that is probably the most valuable lesson that I learned from my father.

Because I couldn't read or write very well, I never looked to science and books for my answers. I figured out things myself and came to my own conclusions. I had very logical thinking and a lot of common sense. I questioned

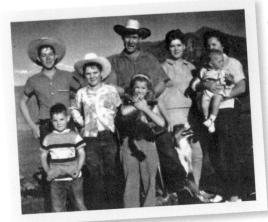

Gary, the tallest boy standing on the far left; Nancy, standing to the right of their father.

everything and was always searching for answers. My intention was to live my life in the mountains and never become part of the "cement world," as it appeared to me. I was very self-sufficient and happy in my environment as long as I had my horses.

My debilitating logging accident in 1973 put me on a very unfamiliar path. Confined to a wheelchair for life, according to the medical prognosis; losing everything, including my family; and after three failed suicide attempts, it became obvious that I was being forced to find a way to live with my pain and misery.

Venturing down an unknown path into science and research was something that had never entered my mind. But that is the very path that has become my passion and has enabled me to accomplish the seemingly impossible: to walk again, to learn to read and write better as an adult, to discover the healing power of essential oils, to formulate supplements with essential oils, and to build my own network marketing company that has grown from a little mom and pop business into a global enterprise with farms and distilleries in different countries around the world—the only company in the world with a Seed to Seal foundation and tens of thousands of members carrying the message of God's healing oils to the far corners of the earth.

I entered the world of healing by default, wanting to heal my own body. I was definitely challenged beyond the little education I had and my exposure to life in general, but I was challenged with a vengeance to understand the human body and to help others as they came to me asking how I was able to get out of the wheelchair and walk again.

Many said it was a miracle. Yes, it was a miracle, but I also knew there was a scientific answer, an answer founded on good nutrition, a strong body, unbending constitution, and unstoppable determination.

I thought a lot about my childhood, especially about my mother. Why was she always sick? Why didn't she like the bread she baked? Why was my father so frustrated when she continued to cook with white sugar against his wishes?

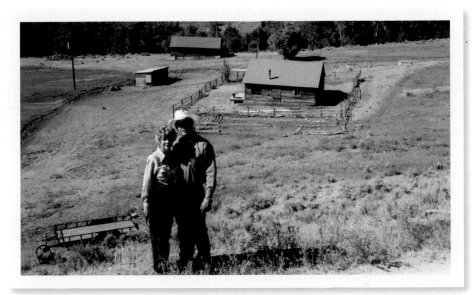

Gary shows Mary the old homestead in Challis, where he grew up.

Mother became addicted to sugar when she was a little girl growing up in the city of Idaho Falls. She ate sugar with and on everything. When we went to visit Grandma and Grandpa, I remember the bowl of white sugar sitting on the table; and when they came to visit us, mother always put a bowl of sugar on the table for them.

Even as a little boy, I could never understand why they ate that stuff. I was different—a non-conformist—the rebellious spirit—the kid with his head in the clouds. Sometimes I felt like the "black sheep" because I felt so different from all of my siblings. I grew up in poverty and had nothing except for the laughter from everyone making fun of us. I wanted something better. I wasn't going to live my adult life—my own life—in poverty, and I never wanted to be sick like my mother. I had visions and ideas, and I daydreamed all the time of what it could be like—and that often got me into trouble in school. The teacher was always telling me to quit daydreaming. I never believed God sent us here to live in sickness and poverty. I was always asking, "Why is Mother sick and why do we live like this?"

I was only five years old when my mother began to show signs of arthritis. She was barely 26 years old when she started complaining about how her hands hurt at night. She was like a weather station, and I knew when the storms were coming by the intensity of her pain. Her knuckles would swell and get stiff, and she would complain about how her body ached.

I always wanted to help her but didn't know how. I would sit with her at night and rub her hands, and she would comment on how much it helped and told me that she wanted me to do well in school and become a doctor because I had healing hands. "No, Mother," I would say, "I just want to be a cowboy like Dad."

My father was always asking for ideas that might help her because when he took her to the doctors in Salmon, Idaho, they just wanted to give her pain pills and anti-inflammatory medicine.

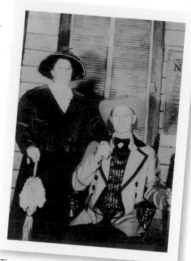

"Tin-type" photo of Gary's parents, Dolly and Donald Young.

Dad took mother to Dr. Milton P. Nelson, a naturopath, who lived in Blackfoot, Idaho, who diagnosed her with hypoglycemia, candida, allergies, and inflammation. Dad didn't care much about what they called these maladies; he just wanted to know what to do to help her.

In 1957 Dad attended a lecture given by a medical doctor, who said white sugar was like a poison that depleted the body of vitamins and minerals. He said that it was just a useless, refined starch and carbohydrate that formed toxic acids that went to the brain and affected the nervous system and was the beginning of degenerative diseases.

Was this white sugar that Mother liked so much really the beginning of her degenerative diseases? That must have been quite a wake-up call for Dad because he came home on fire and said, "No more sugar in the house; we are going to use honey from now on."

However, my father did not know about the high glycemic index of honey, which burns at 110, and that white sugar, regardless of its toxic effect, burns at 86. Mother tried the honey, but every time she ate it, she would go into a hypoglycemic dive that I am sure contributed to her depression, not knowing at that time that she also had low thyroid and low estrogen, something the doctors did not bother to check in those days, at least not in the little farming town of Salmon, Idaho.

In 1958, when mother was expecting again, Dad took her for a check-up to the doctor who had delivered a couple of her other children. He mentioned the diagnosis that Dr. Nelson had made, and Dr. Blackadore called Dr. Nelson a "quack doctor" and said there was no such a thing as candida or hypoglycemia and that they were just quack diseases fabricated by chiropractors and naturopaths to bilk money out of their patients. If they were just imaginary diseases, why did she usually bloat after eating a meal? Why did her joints hurt so much, and why was she constantly tired? None of the doctors had any answers.

Today, hypoglycemia and candida are both metabolic conditions for which doctors prescribe medications. Imagine, prescriptions for "quack diseases." Mother was given a pill that gave her terrible migraine headaches, increased her depression, and made her even more fatigued to where she could hardly get out of bed during the day. She was on and off painkillers for many years and, finally, never stopped taking them.

Shortly after my second sister was born, mother started to put on weight and could not get it off, no matter how hard she worked in the field, the garden, washing clothes in the old tub with the scrub board, and carrying buckets of water to the wood-burning stove in the cabin.

Her low thyroid and low estrogen increased her weight gain, and the depression seemed to increase her craving for more sugar, which led to a lower thyroid, that led to leaky gut syndrome, that led to allergies.

I have since learned that the capacity of the liver is limited, and a daily intake of refined sugar soon makes the liver expand like a balloon. When the liver is saturated to maximum capacity, the excess glycogen is returned to the blood in the form of fatty acids, which are taken to every part of the body and stored in the most inactive areas: the belly, the buttocks, the breasts, and the thighs.

From there, the fatty acids spread to the active organs such as the heart and kidneys, causing the organs to slow down and their tissues to start to degenerate and turn to fat. The entire body is affected, the blood pressure starts to drop, and symptoms of hypoglycemia start to appear.

Refined sugar has a staggering effect on brain function; and when eaten daily, the good bacteria cannot resist and eventually die off, leaving us vulnerable to many diseases like hypoglycemia, fibromyalgia, candida, gluten sensitivities, celiac disease, etc.

If my mother had eaten the honey, she would have at least been ingesting the vitamins, minerals, and enzymes that would have digested in the gut, even though the honey spiked the glucose levels. But she didn't. She continued to eat white sugar and white bread, and her immune system continued to break down. Her thyroid function decreased and her weight increased. Her joints hurt more, her puffy face became puffier, and eventually she was diagnosed with rheumatoid arthritis.

She was so fatigued and depressed and became so intolerant of the cold that she would stay inside all winter except to go out on Sunday to church. The worse she felt, the worse she ate. The more depressed she became, the worse the allergies and the worse the arthritis. It was a vicious cycle and horrible to watch. She was caught in a web, and no one could help her because no one understood what the root cause was.

The cycle is either one of health or one of misery. You cannot have a healthy gut without a healthy thyroid, and you cannot have a healthy thyroid without a healthy gut.

The summer before I started school in 1954, we were driving to Salmon to sell our cream to the creamery. Dad made the trip every month and would use the money to buy food and supplies for the ranch.

This was a big event for my older sister, my younger brother, and me because we rarely traveled anywhere else than to our little town of 650 people, 13 miles from our ranch; and we could only travel when the road was dry, since it was all dirt. When it rained, we couldn't drive because of the mud. In the wintertime, we were snowed in for three months at a time; and when the spring thaw started, we were still land locked because we didn't have a four-wheel drive to get through the mud.

Many times my father would ride his horse out to another ranch 5 miles away and catch a ride to town to get supplies. In the winter when we were snowed in for three months, Dad would snowshoe out to the neighbors to get a ride into town.

Driving to a big city like Salmon that was 78 miles from our farm, with a population of 3,000, was a great adventure for us. After we sold the cream, we went shopping and bought our supplies, had a picnic in the park by the river, and then headed for home.

While driving, we came upon two large boxes approximately 4 x 3 feet sitting in the road that apparently had fallen off of a freight truck. When we stopped to move them off the road, we discovered they were full of different cold cereals like Kellogg's Corn Flakes® and Rice Krispy's®. The other box was full of all kinds of chips that we had never seen before. This was our first introduction to processed foods and packaged cereals that were eaten cold.

All of us were kind of curious about the cold cereal; but after one bowl, I didn't want any more. I thought it was tasteless and unsatisfying, and it left me feeling hungry. I didn't feel any strength or energy from this strange food and preferred my elk steak and my hot cracked wheat cereal, which were the hearty breakfasts that we normally ate. My siblings seemed to enjoy the cold cereal more, and Mother really liked the corn flakes because they didn't upset her stomach like the cracked wheat cereal did. So cold cereal in milk became somewhat of a ritual almost every night until it was gone, but Dad certainly wasn't going to buy any more.

It was easy to see why people liked it. There was no preparation nor clean up, except for the bowel and spoon. How easy it would be to eat like that—like the fast food of today.

We still had to milk the cows morning and night to get the milk that "tasted so good on the flaky cereal." But I preferred my milk on hot cracked wheat. Grinding the wheat was a big chore, but mother's freshly baked bread and cinnamon rolls were worth it. It was just so sad that there was no enjoyment for Mother to do the baking.

I will never forget watching her as she kneaded the bread; her hands ached so much she would cry, until one day she said to my father that she couldn't do it anymore. She developed a rash on her hands, and sometimes her fingertips would swell and crack and bleed when she kneaded the bread.

Mother baked bread every weekend, so we would have it for our school lunches; but by the time I was in Grade 3, she was baking less and less; and when my father asked her why she was not baking bread, she would say to him, "Just pick up a couple of loaves at the store when you go to town for supplies, and get me a loaf of that white bread."

At the age of nine, my older sister Nancy took over the responsibility of making the bread. She took over many other responsibilities as well, since mother was in bed so much of the time.

My father could not understand why my mother was allergic to the wheat we grew on the ranch; it seemed so healthy and no one else in the family was sick. This was before the final hybridization of modern wheat took place in 1955 and entered the commercial market soon after. We never bought seed from anywhere else. We just replanted seeds from what we produced each year and therefore had no exposure to the wheat seed of today.

As I grew older, I continued watching my mother's joints slowly swell as the arthritis created deformity in her fingers. The pain in her hips, shoulders, and back was often so intense that she would cry at night.

She often ate cornmeal because she could handle that without having any acid or heartburn. The corn we grew was not a hybrid, and the wheat we grew

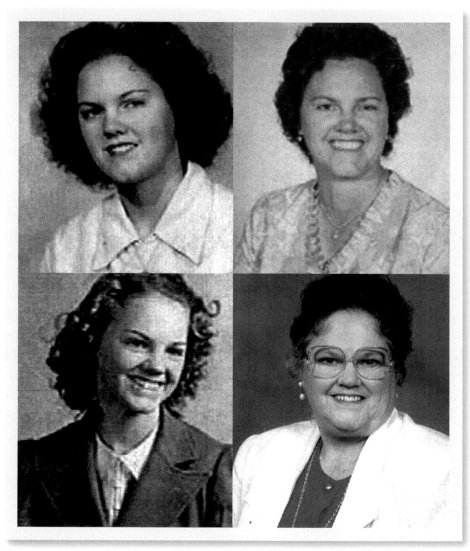

Dolly Adrienne Young. April 27, 1928 - October 12, 2010

was a second-generation hybrid with 28 chromosomes, not the 42 of today. Our wheat grew 4 feet tall, and we cut it with horses, shocked it in the field, and threshed it when it was germinating and the enzymes were active.

Mother couldn't eat anything she baked because of the damage done to her digestive system because of her sugar consumption that probably caused her to have arthritis, candida, and hypoglycemia. She had destroyed her natural intestinal flora and was not producing enough digestive enzymes.

The white bread, devoid of nutrients and made from some kind of processed wheat and bleached with chemicals, had a gluten she could not digest and that destroyed the natural bacteria in the gut that supported her immune and hormonal systems.

My mother had severe pain all through her muscles, ligaments, and joints; and the doctors still couldn't find any reason for it. As I look back, I can see that the pain she demonstrated was just like what people refer to today as fibromyalgia.

Mother lived her entire life with these problems. She seemed to have the symptoms of multiple diseases that the medical establishment did not recognize then; and had they diagnosed the diseases, she would have been taking many medications.

She continued eating in her same destructive way, and for the last 20 years of her life, she was 100 pounds overweight and lived in pain 24/7, even with the pain medication she took.

Watching my mother suffer throughout my youth and not knowing what to do caused a burning curiosity in me to discover answers. I wanted so much to help her, but those answers were yet to come in my future. I knew that there were answers and solutions, and I was going to keep looking and asking until I found them.

Because people can't find answers, they often live with symptoms as just a normal part of life, as common as drinking water. Fibromyalgia is commonly talked about with its symptoms, discomfort, and pain, although some doctors still call it a fad disease, simply because it is hard to diagnose.

More research and education is needed to change the attitude of our scientific community. We need them to recognize that the social and mental dysfunction and neurological behavioral problems are being caused primarily, if not entirely, by the chemicals, toxins, processed foods, and glutens from hybrid grains, etc., whether from eating, breathing, drinking, or applying topically. The human body was not created to digest and assimilate these processed foods and man-made compounds, no matter how we try to justify it.

I have spent the last 30 years of my life in research and discovery, wanting to learn about how to take care of the human body naturally—God's way, without the chemicals and toxins of our modern world. When I was able to walk again, I made a commitment to help others by sharing what I discovered and experienced. My greatest joy is in knowing that someone has been helped with the knowledge that I have shared.

Gary discovers einkorn while conducting research in Azerbaijan in 2001.

CHAPTER I

My Quest to Find Einkorn

When you are a kid, it is amazing how everything seems so big; but as you grow up, those things become smaller. This was the case with wheat that I shocked in the field as a boy. As I thought about those boyhood days, I realized that as an 8- to 10-year-old boy, I was around 38 to 42 inches tall and could stand upright inside the shocks. But as a young adult, the wheat was different at only 14 to 18 inches tall. What happened? There could not have been that much shrinkage over the last 30 years.

I was very fortunate to attend Cairo University at various times from 1991 through 1994 to study bio-chemistry and chemical analysis of essential oils with Professor Dr. Radwan Farag. On the weekends I would catch the cattle train to Upper Egypt and visit the ruins, tombs, pyramids, and all that Upper Egypt offered.

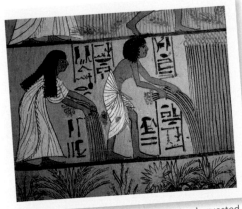

Egyptian hieroglyph showing grain being harvested.

I was fascinated with the reliefs and hieroglyphs on the walls, especially the ones depicting the harvest of the grains. The carvings were usually life-size or bigger and quite proportionately accurate, but the reliefs of the harvesting of the grains were very nonproportional, I thought. But my analytical curiosity prompted me to ask, "If the reliefs are accurate, then their grains were certainly a lot taller than our grains." This is how our wheat looked when I was a boy.

I can remember, 30 plus years later, when I was five years old and in the field with my father harvesting the long shafts of amber grain. Prior to harvest, the head of the wheat reached to the height of a man's chin (about 4 to 4½ feet high).

I wondered what might have caused it to change.

MY EARLY YEARS

I thought back to when I was a little boy when my dad was harvesting our oats and wheat in the early '50s. We did all of our harvesting with horses and an old binding machine that had a reel that swept the stalks back onto the cutter head; and when it cut them, they fell onto the canvas to be bundled.

I can clearly remember that sometimes the seed-laden heads of wheat were actually swept sideways to carry the stalks up between canvas rollers and onto the tying table, where the string was knotted and the bundles were pushed out onto the cradle that carried them through the field until three or four bundles tripped the cradle and released them, making rows of bundles.

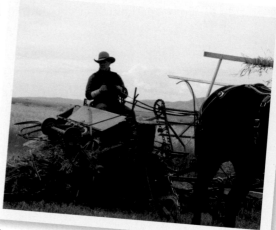

My sister Nancy and I picked up the wheat bundles and stood several of them together like a teepee. They were so tall that they towered over our heads. "Shocking the grain," as it was called, gave the kernels time to mature and start the enzyme activation process prior to threshing. As kids, we had so much

Gary shows the type of equipment his family used to harvest wheat when he was growing up.

fun playing cowboys and Indians hiding inside the "wheat teepees." This definitely wouldn't work with the dwarf 14-inch-tall wheat of today.

We always cut the stalks while they were slightly green and the kernels were firm, which was referred to as the soft dough stage, not when they were totally yellow and hard. When we bit into the kernel, the white liquid inside would squeeze out like a paste. We chewed the kernels all day long because they were so sweet and tasty, whether it was wheat or oats. Chewing the kernels was like having something to snack on all day while we were working in the field.

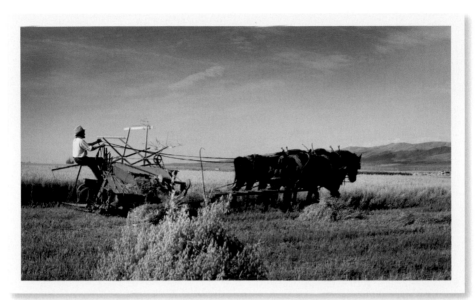

Harvesting oats with a three-horse hitch at the Mona, Utah, farm, as Gary did growing up on the family ranch in Challis, Idaho.

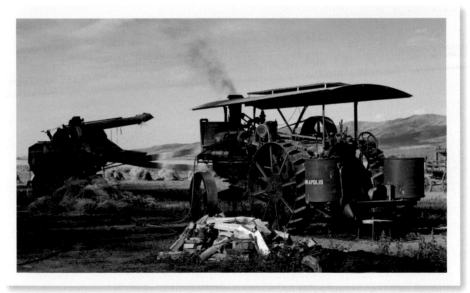

Old threshing machine powered by a steam engine at the Mona, Utah, farm.

At age 12, my job was to drive the team of horses that were harnessed three abreast on the binder to cut the wheat and oats. I loved driving the team; it made me feel so much older, especially watching my younger siblings walking behind to shock the 4- to 5-feet-high shafts of wheat.

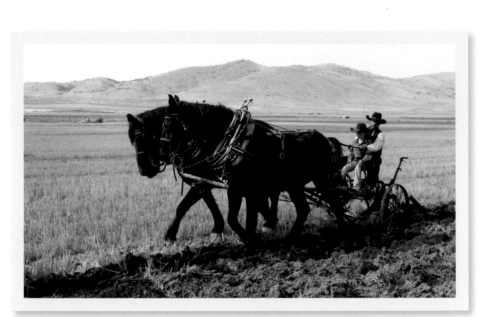

Gary demonstrates at the Mona, Utah, farm how, as a boy, he plowed the field after the wheat harvest to get ready for planting seed for next year's crop.

We left the "grain teepees" standing in the field for 7 to 10 days, during which time the stalks turned from green to a deep yellow that faded just before we loaded them onto the wagons and transported them to the big threshing machine. After threshing, we hauled the wheat kernels to our granary and stored them for our use.

Grinding the grain was tedious with the big hand grinder. Nancy and I would stand on a 3-inch by 12-inch by 4-foot plank to which the grinder was bolted. The kernels were dumped into the head of the hopper, and my father turned the big wheel and ground the grain into cracked cereal that was sometimes cooked for breakfast and sometimes cooked for dinner. At night, after the milking was done, my father changed the stones in the grinder to make finer flour for mother to bake into her beautiful bread.

I never knew what it was like to eat store-bought bread until I was much older, and it certainly did not resemble anything like mother's wood-fired, oven-baked bread. As the children grew older, Mother had Dad buy bread more often when he went to town. I called that bread "cardboard" because that is what it tasted like, and I wasn't going to eat it. I still relished the home-made bread that Nancy baked when mother was no longer able to bake because of the pain in her hands.

What happened to our wheat of yesteryear? When and why did it change? What is the difference between the wheat of today and the wheat I grew up harvesting with my father?

When the family farm in the Snake River Valley near Blackfoot, Idaho, was sold and my father moved to the mountains in Challis, he took our seeds of wheat, oats, and barley with him and planted the grains on our little ranch in the mountains in the late 1940s. It was the same seed that had been grown by his father during the 1920s, the seed crop that carried over each year for the next year's crop. It was the same seed that we planted and harvested every year that fed our family, even after I left home in 1967.

My father sold the ranch in 1972 and moved my mother and my younger siblings to Canada on my homestead while looking for a ranch to buy. He didn't intend to grow wheat and oats anymore, and so he didn't take any seed with him. Naturally, he didn't know anything about hybridized wheat, so he was perfectly happy to buy the local wheat, which he could grind into flour. What we were buying then is hard to say, but it wasn't like the beautiful wheat from the ranch in Challis.

THE WORLD NEEDS MORE FOOD

The demand was growing for more food globally, and wheat appeared to be the commodity that would feed millions of people.

Scientists started looking for ways to increase the wheat yield that eventually led to more hybridizing of more grains. A Nobel Peace Prize was even awarded in 1970 to Dr. Norman Borlaug for his discoveries in hybridizing wheat.

The modern combine made harvesting and threshing a one-time process, so the wheat could go immediately to the granary, making harvesting easier and faster and reducing the cost to the farmer.

But did anyone think about the damage to the wheat? Now there wasn't time for it to germinate, no time to activate the enzymes. The fact that the wheat became difficult to digest, rendering many nutrients unusable, did not seem to be a concern to anybody. Faster production, higher yield, and more money were hailed as a great triumph for the farmers and the brokers. No one could imagine the misery that was about to emerge in new diseases and undiagnosed symptoms. The unsuspecting public was about to become the victim of the new era of food production, a new type of food poisoning.

The process of hybridizing grains has been evolving for a long time. However, modern wheat with its super gluten, super starch, and super drug, which makes it such an addictive carbohydrate, did not come until after 1955, and the first commercial grains and flours started coming on the commercial market shortly thereafter.

If it takes 5 to 10 years for food sensitivities to develop in older people and 20 to 25 years in younger people, someone who was 20 years old in 1960 eating hybridized wheat would be 45 years old 25 years later and starting to develop gluten and food sensitivities in the form of allergies that first manifest perhaps as an irritable bowel condition that might be diagnosed as Crohn's disease, only later to be identified as celiac disease.

In Dr. William Davis's book *Wheat Belly,* he discusses dwarf wheat, explaining that "modern strains of *Triticum aestivum* express a higher quantity of genes for gluten proteins that are associated with celiac disease."[1]

MY SEARCH

So here I was in Egypt, taking photos of the reliefs and saying to myself, "This looks like the wheat we used to grow when I was a kid in the mountains in Idaho." My curiosity seemed to overtake me, and my research became a very clear path of discovery. I became fascinated with the stories of the Hunzakut people in northern Hunza Land and flew there in 1995 to see if I could learn their secrets of longevity.

As Mary and I were driving up the Karimabad Valley into Hunza Land in mid-September, we noticed people down along the river harvesting the wheat by hand. The men were cutting with big scythes, and the women were walking behind, scooping up and tying the stalks of grain into bundles. The children were standing them upright into teepees, just like I had done in my childhood. I had not seen grain harvested this way for nearly 40 years, which brought back a lot of memories.

I had the driver stop the car, and I jumped out and raced down the bank into the little field. I had to know what kind of grain they were harvesting. It resembled wheat, but then it kind of looked like barley because the tufts on the head and the hair were much longer; and yet it didn't look like the barley I knew. There was a significant difference, but I wasn't sure what that difference was. It was identified as a wheat, which is called *chittim* (in Hebrew) in the Old Testament, also referred to in many circles as "farro."

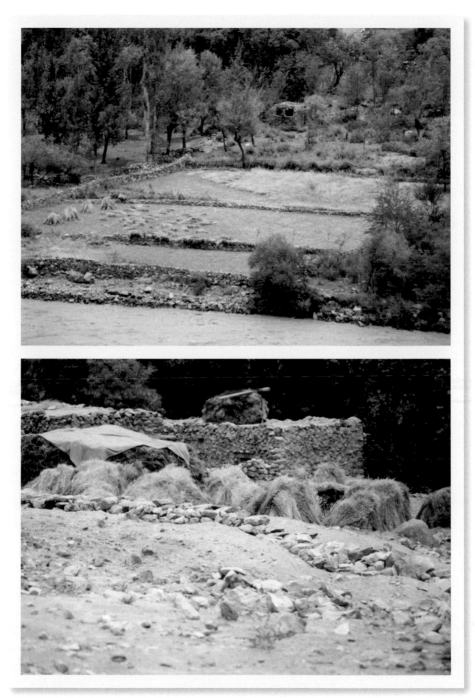

Einkorn cut and shocked, standing in a rocky terrain in Hunza Land in northern Pakistan

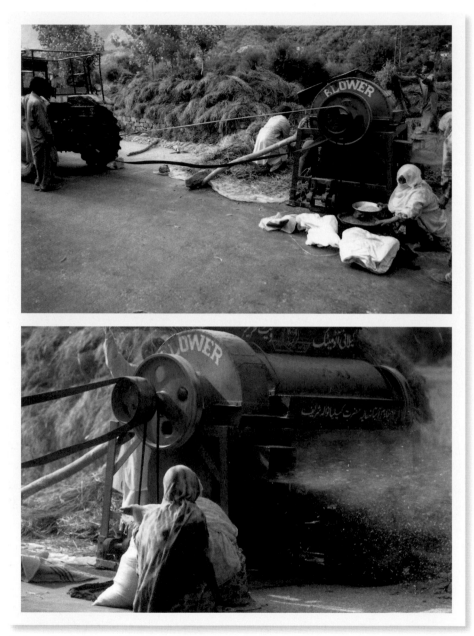

Early mechanized way of threshing einkorn in Pakistan powered by a tractor motor, which turns the belt on the old threshing machine, which then blows out the wheat.

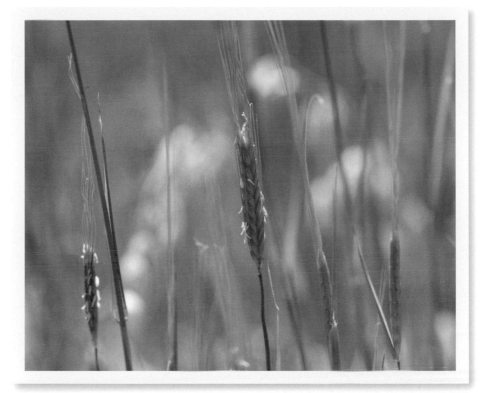

The beginning of einkorn in France

I started searching for einkorn in 1990 and found that it was very difficult to find. I stumbled upon little patches in remote locations (such as Hunza Land of upper Pakistan). I also found it growing on a couple of small farms in Anatolia, Turkey. I even heard that a couple of farmers were growing it on their small farms in Iraq.

In 1999, my quest led me to the east bank of the Jordan River Valley, where I was told einkorn was growing. It was called "farro." For years after, I called it farro, although I heard the word einkorn used occasionally.

A few years later, Jean-Noël, my French farming partner and manager of our farm in France, asked me what I knew about einkorn. I told him I didn't know much but was interested in knowing more, so he told me what he knew. He had located some seed and was eager to plant it. Shortly thereafter, our co-op farmers started growing it, which greatly increased our production, making it possible for commercial use.

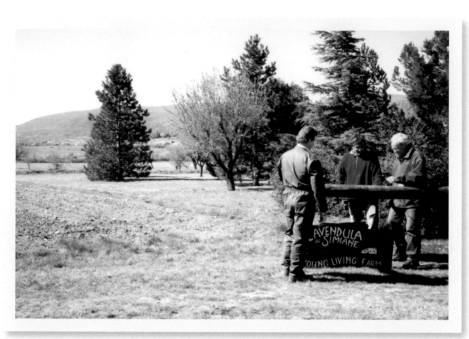

Gary, Jean-Marie, and Jean-Noël discuss expanding einkorn planting on the Young Living farm in France.

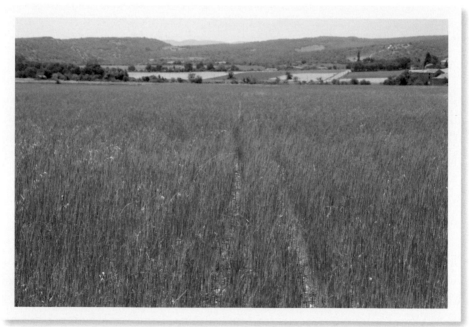

Hearty einkorn growing on the Young Living farm in France.

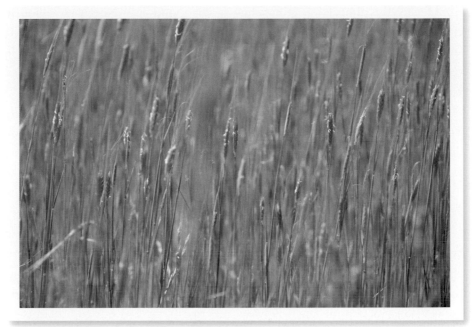

Einkorn thriving on our farm in France, 2014.

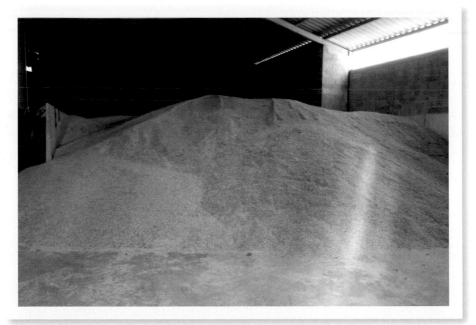

A pile of einkorn after threshing in France.

During this time I was still calling it farro, and Jean-Noël was calling it einkorn; yet we were talking about the same thing. However, in France einkorn is referred to as *petit epeautre*, which means "little spelt," so nicknamed because it resembles spelt, although it is definitely smaller. Most people were as confused as I was. People are still confused between kamut, spelt, farro, and einkorn.

Many indications point to einkorn as being the ancient grain grown in Egypt, the grain stored by Joseph under the reign of Ramses in preparation for the seven years of famine, the same grain that has been growing in Hunza Land for thousands of years. Fascinating possibilities.

It has been five years now since we started growing einkorn on our farm in France, along with several neighbors who wanted to co-op grow with us.

Two years ago we also started growing little test patches of einkorn on our farm in Utah. We planted and harvested this seed again and again until we were able to harvest enough seed to expand our field. Last year we had a very successful small harvest of einkorn; and this year, 2014, we have over 35 acres of einkorn growing on our farm in Utah. Between our two farms and our co-op farms in France, we are growing over 250 acres of einkorn.

We now have enough flour from our farms in France and Utah to start making it available for limited distribution.

ANCIENT EINKORN

Einkorn is considered the ancient grain or the original wheat of man. Its botanical name is *Triticum monococcum* and has the simplest genetic code of all the varieties of wheat with just 1 genome and 14 chromosomes. The stocks are long and slender, and the kernels are oblong and flat looking and are protected by a strong husk or chaff that clings to the kernels. Einkorn grows to be about 4.5 to 5 feet tall with hair-like tassels that easily wave in the wind.

The common wheat of today is called "dwarf wheat" because it grows to be only about 16 inches high. It has double the amount of kernels that are thicker and heavier looking, with very little hair and a soft husk that is easily removed. Modern wheat has 42 chromosomes, which is difficult for the body to digest and can be the beginning of many different physical problems and diseases.

Einkorn is a "hulled" wheat because of its tough husk or chaff, not a "free threshing" wheat like today's durum and dwarf wheats, which have a husk around the grain that is easily loosened and removed by threshing.

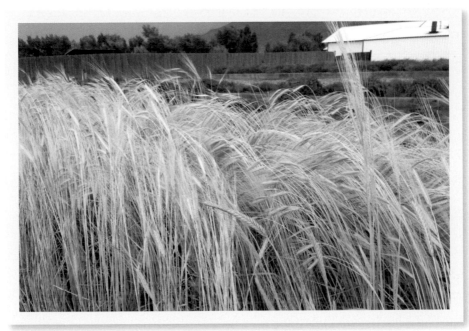
Einkorn growing extremely well on the Young Living farm in Mona, Utah.

The older wheat varieties, einkorn, emmer, and spelt, are called "hulled" wheat because a tough hull or husk clings to the grain and must be removed. One method is to take a bat or stick and beat the dried wheat heads off the shaft. The Roman historian Pliny the Elder (from the 1st century A.D.) wrote about the Etruscans grinding grain in his *Natural History* (Book 4, pages 36-37). "All the grains are not easily broken. In Etruria they first parch [roast slightly] the spelt in the ear, and then pound it with a pestle shod with iron at the end. . . . Throughout the greater part of Italy, however, they employ a pestle that is only rough at the end."

While getting the grain out of hulled wheat like einkorn is more difficult, the tough hull is protective against pests. For this reason, einkorn, emmer, and spelt are easier to grow organically. An Italian conference on hulled wheat reported, "The fact that hulled wheats are mainly grown in mountainous areas today is not simply a result of their isolation; hulled wheats do seem especially resistant to poor soil conditions and a range of fungal diseases."[2]

The two other types of ancient wheat are emmer and spelt; and like einkorn, they are hulled wheats. Emmer is a cross between wild wheat and wild goat

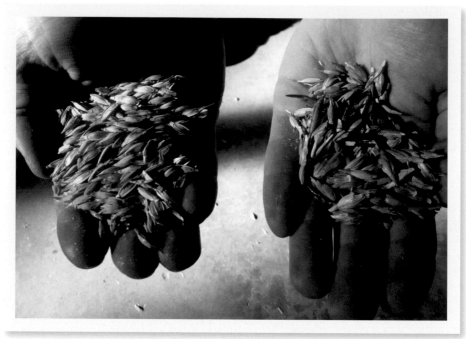

Gary shows einkorn in his right hand, which is lighter, and spelt in his left hand, which is darker. It is easy to see why people have a difficult time telling them apart.

grass called *Aegilops speltoides* and has 28 chromosomes. Spelt is a hybrid of a domesticated wheat like emmer and another wild grass (*Aegilops tauschii*). Spelt (today often called kamut) has 42 chromosomes. Emmer and spelt have *not* been extensively cross-hybridized like dwarf wheat and have developed naturally; there is no evidence that einkorn has been cross-pollinated.

Some writers claim that spelt originated in Asia before bread wheat appeared. But a study shows that European spelt in the Northern Alpine region has allelic variation that came from a restricted growing area, while glutenin alleles between Asian spelt and bread wheat allows a scenario where Asian spelt "originates from the hulled ancestors of bread wheat."[3] This simply means that Asian spelt and European spelt had different origins.

Einkorn very well could have grown in multiple locations, similar to the fir tree that grows from Alaska to Mexico and the blue spruce tree that grows from New Brunswick, Canada, to northern Arizona. It is not just isolated to one single location. It would seem logical that the ancient caravaners carried einkorn seed to many different places, and it would have been grown to feed people living in diverse places.

The Fertile Crescent

My research and that of other researchers (a consensus of archaeologists) is that einkorn (German for "one korn" or grain) was first domesticated in the northern and eastern parts of the Fertile Crescent, along a region of the Euphrates/Tigris River system called Mesopotamia.

The Fertile Crescent encompasses Israel, including Gaza, all the way up through Tel Aviv to Lebanon and Syria, then makes an arch and follows the Tigris/Euphrates River system all the way down, encompassing the southern part of Turkey, Anatolia (Asia Minor), which takes in a great deal of Iran and Iraq.

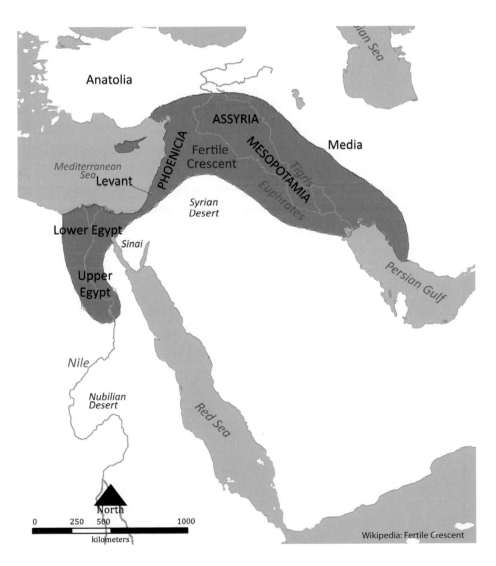

Wikipedia: Fertile Crescent

That was the richest farming and agricultural area in the ancient world and was one of the first areas where plants were domesticated. Many researchers believe that einkorn was man's first domesticated grain.

Some archaeologists believe that early civilization that first developed in Mesopotamia started around 12,000 to 10,000 B.C. These people established the first writing systems and were the first to construct buildings out of materials other than sticks, mud, and animal skins. They made different types of mortar by mixing together liquefied crushed grains, straw chaff, and mud. In some cases goat milk was even added to help create a dough-like consistency so that the mud had a more binding effect. Even camel dung and cow manure were mixed into this mortar to help it dry and harden.

In the Arabian countries where frankincense resin was available, people would crush the resin and heat it in vats. With the temperatures of the Arabian Desert reaching a scorching 120 degrees Fahrenheit and the sun's heat further increasing the temperature by 10 or 20 degrees, the frankincense would stay emulsified and moist in the liquid. The warm and pliable frankincense could then be removed from the water and used for a variety of applications, including use in a cast around a camel's (or human's) broken leg. After the cast was molded, layers of frankincense resin were put on it to seal the injury from moisture and infection, just like a synthetic resin today is put on a fabric for building a canoe.

The knowledge that the ancient people had was phenomenal, despite their limited education. As various rulers conquered different regions, they would see villagers making bricks in different ways, constructing buildings, farming, etc., and then take that knowledge back to their country.

It is possible that barley grew in southern Mesopotamia and that einkorn grew in upper Mesopotamia in the Anatolia regions of Turkey. As different armies were invading neighboring countries, the warriors traveled back and forth taking different grains home with them.

Einkorn and barley might not have been indigenous to northern India or China. So how did they get there? They likely went with the caravan traders who were traveling west to exchange goods or traversing the great Silk Road from Rome to China. The Chinese developed the silkworm farms and created the exotic fabric of silk, for which the demand grew dramatically. As silk was transported to many countries, so were many other goods, including seeds and other agricultural commodities.

Ancient Commerce

It has been thought that around 1800 B.C., travelers seeking adventures in foreign lands began to explore the regions around the Tigris and Euphrates rivers. Many people were interested in visiting the regions because they had read or heard about them in the accounts of the Greek, Roman, and other writers who wrote and talked about their expeditions.

Military forces that traveled to conquer generally took a scribe to record the events of the war. That scribe would also record the events and culture of the people they warred against. This information was written in different forms and in different ways, and the stories evolved as they were handed down.

We know that caravans brought frankincense and myrrh up from southern Arabia, present day Oman, across the Empty Quarter coming through Jabrin to Gerrha, and loaded the resins onto ships that sailed the Persian Gulf to the mouth of the Euphrates/Tigris River system. Those merchants were trading for all kinds of merchandise. Einkorn wasn't growing in Oman, but it could have. Is it possible that the caravaners *traded* for einkorn because it was considered a valuable, life-sustaining food and because the seed could be replanted every year? Many researchers believe that ancient einkorn is the most nutritious grain that has ever been grown in the world and credit it as the foundation of modern civilization, which could not exist without it.

The story of Joseph in the Bible and the seven years of feast and famine took place about 2000 B.C. Some people say that the grain written about might have been kamut, but that isn't possible because kamut is a hybrid. Many archeologists believe that kamut did not exist until about 2,000 years ago.

Einkorn seeds were carried thousands of miles all the way from India to China to Pakistan and down to Ethiopia in Africa. They were even carried as far south as Marib, the ancient capital of what is known as Yemen today. The Hadhramut, as it was called then, was where the Queen of Sheba is said to have brought einkorn back after the King Solomon caravan of 980 B.C. and planted it in Yemen.

Some people think that thousands of years ago, agriculture began its earnest development in the Middle East and perhaps as far east as China. What is interesting is that researchers have found evidence of einkorn in central Mexico, in the ancient pyramids of farming communities that evolved around the same period of time in the Andes and in Nicaragua. Large fields with these wild grains are still found in Anatolia today.

Filming of "The One Gift" documentary, depicting camel caravan traders arriving in Petra, Jordan, an ancient trading center.

Early Cultivation and Hybridization

How did the first hybridization of wild wheat and goat grass take place? Perhaps one farmer in the Mesopotamian Valley was growing wild wheat because it grew well in the lowlands where he lived and was easy to harvest. But on the other side of the river, a farmer grew wild grass for his goats. Hence, the nickname "wild goat grass."

One day the Euphrates River flooded, and the wild goat grass seeds that were on the ground washed into the fields where the wild wheat grew. There probably wasn't a great deal of difference between them thousands of years ago. The farmers weren't picky about it, and they weren't trying to certify their seed; they only grew and harvested it for feeding their family and animals. So the two wild grains grew together and cross-pollinated naturally.

I have watched Idaho tansy seed be carried by the floodwaters of the Palouse River downstream and wash out onto a farmer's field in high season; and guess what: where tansy didn't grow last year, it grows this year.

In ancient times, people didn't spray their crops, they just let the crops and weeds grow together. This might be how the wild wheat and wild goat grass cross-pollinated and became the first hybridized grain, known as emmer, a new strain of wheat.

Somewhere in that process, the hybridization altered the genomes and DNA. Emmer wheat, as it is known today, added 14 more chromosomes to the 14 it already had to now total 28.

Then emmer seeds cross-pollinated with other wild grass seeds, and yet another hybridized wheat sprang up. This time the 14 chromosomes from the goat grass were added to the 28 chromosomes of emmer wheat, producing the hybrid wheat we call spelt, which has 42 chromosomes.

Emmer and another grass were cross-pollinated to produce a hybrid with 3 genomes (instead of 1) and became the parent of the hybrid "dwarf" wheat of today. Three sets of DNA connected together with a never-been-seen-before genomic construction capable of producing never-been-seen-before proteins.

Is eating food from this "natural" DNA-spliced monstrosity healthy?

It is believed that different grains such as barley, einkorn, rye, chickpeas, and legumes were being cultivated in what is now Syria, Lebanon, Israel, and Palestine around 10,000 years ago. The first evidence of barley was found in the Jordan Valley dated at about that same time period.

The first ancient variety of grain I found growing was in the Jericho Valley. The earliest levels of excavation at Jericho indicate that people who lived there collected seeds of cereal grasses from rocky crags around the valleys and planted them in the fertile soils near the villages. Archaeologists who excavated to the very beginning of the city of Jericho found a number of storage jars of charred grain from the last Canaanite city, suggesting it was conquered at harvest time and then burned.

Mesopotamia was originally very swampy in some areas and dry in others, which suggests that they certainly could have started an irrigation system. A lot of things happen just by nature. For example, people might plant the field, it gets dry, a flash flood comes, the field gets irrigated naturally; and they discover that after the flash flood, the field grew two or three times more quickly and effectively. So then they begin to carry water from the river and put it on their crops. In the very beginning, a lot of irrigation was done using buckets and bucket brigades packing water to the fields and pouring it around the plants.

Many people likely migrated with their families, their seeds, and their animals and moved to a new location to replant and reestablish their farms and fields. As the camel caravans transported many different goods, grains became well-known as commodities that were worth money and suitable for trading.

Archaeological evidence and research from carbon dating of seeds takes this ancient grain back perhaps 10,000 or 11,000 years. By using DNA fingerprinting, it was found that the first domestication was in the areas of the Karacadağ Mountains near Diyarbakir in southwestern Turkey, northern Syria and Iran, and northwest Iraq.[4,5]

Ötzi, the Iceman

One of the most fascinating archaeological finds was the September 1991 discovery of the body of a man, approximately 5,000 years old, who had been frozen in ice in the Ötzal Alps above 10,000 feet on the border between Austria and Italy. Ötzi, the "Iceman" from the Tyrolean Alps, was discovered by two Austrian hikers, who stumbled across his frozen remains. They were shocked to discover that his body was very much intact, even though two-thirds of it had been exposed for some time. His clothing, tools, artifacts of survival and war, and fire-making tools were found on and around his body.

From Wikipedia: "Analysis of Ötzi's intestinal contents showed two meals (the last one consumed about eight hours before his death), one of chamois meat, the other of red deer and herb bread. Both were eaten with grain as well as roots and fruits. The grain from both meals was a highly processed einkorn wheat bran, quite possibly eaten in the form of bread."[6]

This is an amazing find. It is very possible, however, that emmer, spelt, or einkorn could have been in Ötzi's stomach because all three grains existed at that time.

Ancient Grains

Traveling from the Alps to Egypt, we find more documentation of ancient grains. Along with the reliefs and writings on the walls in the temples and tombs in Egypt, there are many depictions of grain and bread making. However, we cannot determine specifically which grain it is. When King Tutankhamen's tomb was opened in 1922, not only did archaeologists find the alabaster vases that had contained essential oils (the oils were stolen by grave robbers), but they found baskets of grain that could have been einkorn, emmer, or khorasan grain, which is now called kamut.

Is it possible that different varieties of grains grew in ancient Egypt? Kamut likes a little gentler farming environment, whereas einkorn prefers a rougher, rugged-type terrain, where a lot of other grains won't grow. Einkorn can withstand hot and cold temperatures, while kamut is a little more fragile and likes temperatures a little more consistent, like you see in Egypt, although because of the extreme mid-summer heat, I question whether kamut would survive. However, from my experience in growing einkorn and seeing fields of it growing in different areas of the world, einkorn is definitely more suitable for the rugged soil and heat of Egypt.

THE ANCIENT PROCESS OF GROWING WHEAT

Seeds from these grains ripen (mature) over a period of three weeks, and someone using a blade and a sickle could harvest about 2 pounds of grain per hour.

I am sure from trial and error that farmers knew they could not cut the grain when it was ripe because the impact of the scythe on the stalk as you cut it would shake loose the wheat grains, especially if it were dry. Gathering all those small kernels would be very difficult, so they likely discovered that by cutting the wheat stalks while they were immature and in an immature stage, they could keep the kernels attached to the head of the wheat stalk.

Hybridized wheat enables modern harvesting to bypass the different stages of development. Today the grain is cut and threshed immediately, so it has no time to go through that maturing stage to germinate and develop the enzymatic activity needed later for digestion. Wheat is harvested for man's convenience, not

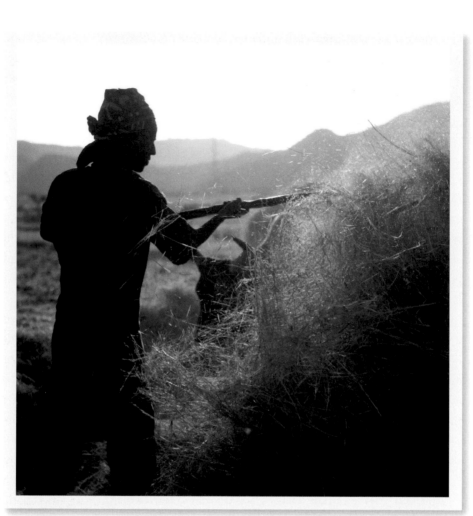

Harvesting einkorn in Ethiopia today.

for maximizing health benefits.

In ancient times farmers would not have understood the science of harvesting wheat, but they must have known that the wheat was more health-sustaining when it went through all the stages of maturing.

In order for the kernels to mature, they require the moisture and humidity that collects at night to stimulate enzyme activity and promote proper maturation. This increase of enzyme activity within the kernel not only helps the grain reach proper maturation, but it also augments our own natural enzymes when we consume it.

It was easy to see the visible maturation of the stalks as the stems changed color from green to greenish yellow and to completely yellow. The kernels would transform from soft to brittle, and the husks would harden and lose their pliable and flexible structure.

When the husks dried out, the kernels could then break free. Cutting the stalks while slightly green meant the husks were not yet brittle and would not come off easily, and the kernels would not be hard enough to fall from the head.[7]

The wheat kernels (edible seeds or grains) were sometimes threshed (separated from the inedible chaff or husk) by spreading them on a hard surface and letting cattle or donkeys walk over them. I saw this in Ethiopia when I was researching frankincense.

Farmers would also beat the grain with sticks to loosen and dislodge the kernels from both the husk and the head of the wheat. This was only possible if the kernels were mature and fully "ripe."

As an example, I would compare mature wheat to a vine-ripened tomato. Conversely, the modern man-made wheat of today that is harvested green and immature is equivalent to a non-vine-ripened tomato that is red but tastes like cardboard and has the nutritious value of an egg crate.

Harvested, fully mature wheat kernels are also easier to store than other foodstuffs. Once dry, they are easy to keep. Weevils, however, are a problem, but they are easy to remove by screening them out.

Agriculture has allowed men to evolve from a survival hunter-type to more of a domesticated farmer-type. In the process we have transformed wheat from a mature, hardy, nutritionally-dense food into an immature, hot-house, man-made creation with little nutritional benefit.

THE NUTRITIOUS BIBLICAL GRAIN

The Bible's first mention of "wheat" is in Genesis 30:14: "And Reuben went into the days of wheat harvest and found mandrakes in the field and brought them unto his mother Leah."

"Wheat" is the English word, not the Aramaic, Greek, or Hebrew word for "einkorn," the ancient wheat. Einkorn is the German translation for wheat. In the Old Testament the word for "wheat" is *chittah*. There is a lot of speculation about what the correct English word is for einkorn. However, because many of the archeologists and researchers are of European origin, they have chosen to stay with the German translation and call it "einkorn."

Today we use a lot of slang words and common words but not necessarily botanical words. Certainly thousands of years ago, they did not use a botanical identity for talking about grain. But after reviewing a lot of research material related to the translation, it appears that einkorn was known in biblical times as *chittah*, or *chittim*, which is plural for more than one grain.

Strong's Concordance also tells us that the word for "wheat" is *chittah*; and for more than one grain of wheat, the plural word is *chittim*. It is interesting that in German and Hebrew, the root word for wheat means just "one grain."

Many people believe that einkorn was the biblical wheat of ancient times, so we could refer to it as a spiritual food that fed the tribes of Israel.

In the next chapter, we will look at one thing we can document for sure that has changed—hybridization of wheat by man. In the years since that change, it has been the focus of studies showing results no one ever expected. This may be the beginning of the new apocalypse of our modern diseases and undiagnosed symptoms that have been slowly advancing upon the world like an "avenging angel" of sickness and death.

ENDNOTES

1   Davis W, MD. *Wheat Belly*, Rodale, 2011:26.
2   Padulosi S, Hammer K, Heller J, ed. Hulled Wheat. *Proceedings of the First International Workshop on Hulled Wheats,* Castelvecchio Pascoli, Tuscany, Italy, 21-22 July 1995:41.
3   Blatter RHE, et al. About the origin of European spelt (*Triticum spelta* L.): allelic differentiation of the HMW Glutenin B1-1 and A1-2 subunit genes, *Theor Appl Genet.* 2004, 108:360-67.
4   Heun M, et al. Site of Einkorn Domestication Identified by DNA Fingerprinting, *Science,* 14 November 1997:1312-14.
5   Athena Review: *Journal of Archaeology, History, and Exploration.* http://www.athenapub.com/einkorn1.htm.
6   Holden TG. The Food Remains from the Colon of the Tyrolean Ice Man, in Keith Dobney; Terry O'Connor, *Bones and the Man: Studies in Honour of Don Brothwell,* Oxford: Oxbow Books, 2002:35–40.
7   Zadok's Wheat Development Stages. http://www.extension.umn.edu/agriculture/small-grains/growth-and-development/spring-wheat/.

CHAPTER 2

The Decline of Nutrition

"Why me?" is a common complaint. "I don't deserve to have cancer, nor does my mother, nor my wife, nor my father. I don't deserve to have heart disease, diabetes, dementia, celiac disease, etc."

You are right. You don't deserve it, but you developed it with every bite.

MODERN AILMENTS: AN OVERVIEW

It is shocking to think that the decline in nutrition started about 2,000 years ago, and that was probably with the first hybridization of wheat. Some of the early diagnoses were about 1,800 years ago; and there are even scrolls with writings about "sprue," which today is known as celiac disease.

Intestinal disease in India was called sprue and was written about in Sanskrit as early as 15 B.C. Aretaeus, a European author in the 2nd century A.D., coined the term "coeliac" from the Greek word for belly to describe the abdominal distention experienced by people suffering from this condition.

In 1969, Vincent Katelaer, a Dutch physician, described it as "stomatitis aphthous" in his treatise on sprue, which was considered a childhood disease.

Dr. F. Curtis Dohun, from the Medical College of Pennsylvania, stated that wheat gluten can induce common behavioral disturbances in both children and adults who have celiac symptoms and said that wheat gluten may enter the brain and affect the nerve receptor sites.

Other investigators concluded that schizophrenia is more prominent where wheat is a staple grain.

In Toronto, 115 people with celiac were examined and shown to have a high level of diabetes.

In Finland, 110 celiac children under the age of two and 22 children over the age of two showed a higher-than-average incidence of diabetes.

Does gluten have anything to do with infertility? Absolutely! The severe, gluten-caused celiac disease seems to impact reproductivity in women more frequently than in men, judging by the number of studies.

A 2014 study analyzed previous research for women and concluded, "Patients with unexplained infertility, recurrent miscarriage or intrauterine growth restriction were found to have a significantly higher risk of CD [celiac disease] than the general population."[1]

Another study reported on "a case of a woman presenting with primary infertility who on investigation was found to have celiac disease and had a successful conception when on a gluten-free diet for a period of 8 months."[2]

For the men, research shows that ". . . in men with coeliac disease there is a derangement of pituitary regulation of gonadal function."[3] Italian researchers reported, "The male CD patient has a greater risk of infertility and other reproductive disturbances."[4]

Wheat gluten is used in many different ways. Stabilizers, emulsifiers, starches, binders, fillers, and bulking agents are all made from wheat gluten. It is used to prevent shrinkage and moisture loss in cooking. It emulsifies fats and other substances, binds juices, and improves the texture of many foods. It is used as a binder of meat products like sausage, beef, pork, steaks, meat rolls, textured vegetable protein, fish, and meat extenders in packaged meals. Wheat gluten is also used to glaze over foods such as meat patties and sausage and is used as an adhesive to bind batter and breading agents.

Gluten absorbs twice its weight in water for rapidly increasing the yield of many processed foods. It is added to imitation cheese to make it stretch. It is also added to many breakfast cereals—including "non-gluten" cereals made from oats—alcoholic beverages, ice cream, ketchup, mayonnaise, and in some instant coffees. Wheat-free bread is made with gluten to give it more body. Lipstick, eye makeup, toothpaste, and many foundations for cosmetics use wheat gluten as a binder.

The arrival of the Industrial Age and the mechanization of farm equipment increased the cost of farming. Farmers needed to reduce farming costs but yet increase the yield, which was one factor that led to the hybridization of wheat and other grains.

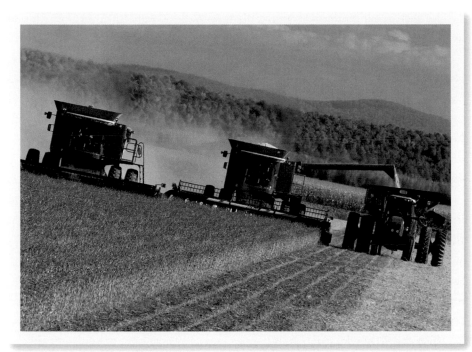
Mechanized harvesting and threshing of today's hybrid wheat.

Next came hybrids, synthetic pesticides, and fertilizers, which further increased the yield but at the cost of introducing toxins into the food supply, killing the enzymes that are so important for digestion and killing the natural microbes in the soil. Then the grains that had fed the world were hybridized and eventually genetically engineered.

OUR FOOD SUPPLY

What has happened to our food supply? Why do so many people have wheat gluten intolerance? Gradually, the idea of gluten intolerance spread like an epidemic—that the body had a genetic defect that possibly caused arthritis, enteritis, schizophrenia, celiac disease, irritable bowel syndrome, gastritis, Crohn's disease, dementia, fibromyalgia, autism, TDD (temper dysregulation disorder), ANS (autonomic nervous system) disorders, bipolar, manic depression, etc., especially since all of these diseases show connections to wheat gluten.

During the last few years, more ailments with animals have entered the sickness arena. The increase of colic in horses has gone up substantially. The study on pig stomach inflammation provides more evidence that would lead us to believe that wheat gluten and genetically modified food are unfit for both animal and human consumption and may cause severe damage to the digestive system.

Modern wheat turns to glucose three times faster than white sugar. Because gluten is a super starch, a super fat, and a super drug, it is very addictive and causes cravings for carbohydrates that increase blood sugar, blood insulin, fat storage, and food intolerances. It decreases hormone-sensitive lipase, which is the fat-burning hormone, so the incidence of overweight and obesity continues to soar.

Each year, research shows us that the number of people with celiac disease and gluten intolerance is increasing, causing people to suffer with food allergies, heartburn, digestive problems, and other maladies. Interestingly, there are many similarities between gluten intolerance, acne, arthritis, osteoporosis, bursitis, rheumatism, and many other afflictions.

Arthritis starts with simple joint pain, stiffness, a weak immune system, frequent colds, the flu, stuffy nose, and head and respiratory congestion three or four times a year. Every time the temperature changes or the wind blows, another cold or sniffle appears; and people say it's because it's allergy season. Then they begin to think they are allergic to pollens and can't live here or can't live there.

We blame everything on the environment around us; and, granted, there is a lot of merit to that. People who are gluten sensitive or have been diagnosed with celiac disease experience joint pain, swelling, and stiffness if they eat foods with wheat gluten. Why? Because wheat gluten does not digest. The super gluten, the super starch, the super drug, and the fermentation they cause creates an acid condition in the body and a lot of inflammation that decreases the body's uptake of oxygen. This creates hypoxia, which is oxygen deprivation in the tissue. Anytime there is oxygen deprivation in the tissue, there is pain.

In the early stages, celiac disease is often confused with and diagnosed as arthritis. Many times people with terrible acne who stop eating gluten foods notice that the acne starts to go away. Many people complain about having muscle stiffness, muscle pain, and joint pain; but an x-ray of the joint indicates there is no irregularity. In some severe cases, an MRI scan will show some inflammation.

Arthritis definitely indicates a possibility of gluten intolerance and fibromyalgia, along with adult autistic behavior. Arthritis is highly inflammatory and affects the neurological system, as well as the musculoskeletal system. Wheat gluten intolerance or celiac disease could easily cause arthritis symptoms.

Rheumatoid arthritis is an autoimmune condition, whereby the body mistakenly sees normal healthy parts of itself as being foreign, causing the body's immune system to attack and try to destroy those "harmful invaders."

In the case of celiac disease, the body responds to the gluten by attacking and destroying the villi that line the small intestine that help the body absorb nutrients. It breaks the villi tight junctions, allowing food particles and gases to enter into the bloodstream that contribute to brain fog and other allergic symptoms that manifest because of the chemical reaction of the toxins in the blood.

Anyone with rheumatoid arthritis is at risk of developing other diseases such as cancer, celiac disease, fibromyalgia, heart disease, etc.

I believe arthritis is not a disease; it is an allergy. If you eliminate the foods to which your body is allergic or intolerant, you will notice that with good enzymes, you will be able to assimilate the minerals that are important to help prevent your body from developing arthritis. You will increase the circulation, the blood flow, and the oxygen into the tissues, which all help to alleviate arthritic symptoms.

More than 3 million Americans have celiac disease, according to the National Digestive Diseases Information Clearinghouse. However, more than 21 million Americans have arthritis, according to the Center for Disease Control and Prevention. Having one increases the risk for having the other.

Over 80 percent of the food that is ingested today is processed and completely devoid of enzymes. How do we replenish the enzymes needed for proper digestion and metabolic function in the digestive tract? How can the body produce the proteins, hormones, vitamins, minerals, etc., that the body needs if the nutrients are not in the food? The body can't—so more symptoms and diseases evolve with fancy names for which the doctors write more prescriptions.

The day will come when these neurological and pathological behaviors and social development problems in our children will become as commonplace as the common cold; and two decades from now, people will say, "Oh, that's just the way it is." At some point autistic conditions will probably become just as commonplace as hypoglycemia, and that day is just about here. If we don't change our habits and ways of eating, our society will be altered forever.

OBESITY

The U.S. Center for Disease Control gave the latest (2011-2012) statistics on weight: 31.1 percent of adults age 20 and older are obese; 69.0 percent of adults age 20 and older are overweight, including those who are obese.[5]

The World Health Organization's website reports that worldwide obesity has nearly doubled since 1980. In 2008, more than 1.4 billion adults, 20 and older, were overweight. Of these, over 200 million men and nearly 300 million women were obese.[6]

Have you ever walked into a smorgasbord or a salad bar and watched people eat? It's like hogs at a trough. Everything imaginable is placed on the plate. The mindset seems to be, "Wow, this smorgasbord is only $12.95, and I'm going to make the most of it. I'm going to eat all that I can and get my money's worth."

First comes the plate with mashed potatoes and gravy, chicken, squash, lasagna, macaroni and cheese, a large white roll, that plastic spread called "butter," and thick jam, all piled up on one plate.

Second is another plate loaded with lettuce, peas, broccoli, beets, carrot shreds, and cottage cheese from the salad bar and even some sprouts because "sprouts are very nutritious."

Third is a drink to wash down all the food; so let's tank up with a tall glass of soda pop with either sugar or aspartame, a known carcinogen, or a "healthy" glass of processed, imitation fruit juice.

Fourth is a trip or two to the dessert bar. The choices are amazing: strawberry, chocolate, vanilla, or a combination of ice cream flavors, yogurt, carrot cake with tons of frosting loaded with sugar, cherry pie, apple pie, apple crisp waiting for the whipped cream to be put on top, and maybe a piece of German chocolate cake or chocolate mousse or some other delicious delicacy. The strawberries, drenched in a sugary syrup, are ready for indulgence with chocolate chip cookies, donuts, and/or cinnamon rolls on the side. Yum!

Sometimes people try a piece of almost every dessert on the dessert bar with no awareness of how the body will feel with all that packed in on top of what they just ate. One plate of food is bigger than the human stomach, but two plates of food with that huge plate of dessert? The poor stomach had to expand three times its normal size to accommodate that one meal for only $12.95. What a deal.

Then as they waddle out of the restaurant to the parking lot, they wonder why they feel sluggish and their head hurts, not daring to look in the mirror on

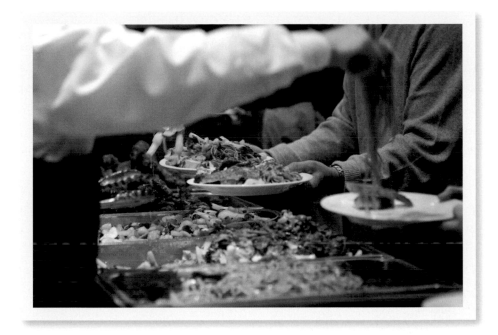

their way out and see those extra 10, 25, or even 100 pounds and wonder where it all came from; "It must be lack of exercise." But then they did give themselves some good nutrition with the salad they ate; too bad it was likely treated with pesticides and chemicals, since none of it was organic.

Are an engorged stomach and obesity caused by overeating? That's a no brainer.

Triathletes Get Fat, Too!

What about the people who exercise daily more than you and I do in a lifetime? What happens to a triathlete who competes in a "Half Ironman" and swims 1.2 miles, bikes 112 miles, and then runs 26.2 miles? Dr. William Davis, author of *Wheat Belly,* writes, "The majority of triathletes adhere to fairly healthy eating habits. Then, why are a third of these dedicated men and women athletes overweight?"[7]

What has changed in the diet that would cause one third of the extreme athletes to be overweight while on an intense training program? Something changed that caused a spike in weight gain and in diseases like diabetes, celiac disease, hypoglycemia, candida, etc. How do we get our health back?

The answer is very simple; we have to change our way of eating.

A DIFFERENT ENVIRONMENT

A high-functioning, autistic 11-year-old girl was brought to me by her parents to see if I had any suggestions that might make her world better. I asked to speak with her alone to see if I could discover what she was feeling. She told me how different she felt when she was with her grandparents in the country instead of being in the apartment in the city. She told me that she had tried to tell her parents how she felt, but they didn't seem to understand what she was trying to say.

She told me that she loved to visit and stay with her grandparents. She had fun with her grandpa working in the garden, and her grandma always made special meals with the food that they grew. She told me that she liked the food a lot better than the frozen food her mother cooked in the microwave at home. Grandma didn't buy any soda pop or sugary cereal. Grandpa raised a few goats and the milk tasted so creamy.

She explained how her grandma taught her to get water out of the well and that it tasted different than the water at home, which had kind of a different smell and a taste she really didn't like.

She said that the longer she stayed with her grandma and grandpa, the better she felt. She could think better and she could speak without stumbling over her words. She said she tried to tell her parents how much happier she was with her grandparents, and they just kind of ignored her. But she knew that as soon as she returned to the city, she began to feel different and things didn't work very well for her.

It was obvious what was happening, but the parents were set in their ways and very unaware of their toxic environment. As I started pointing out these things to the parents, they were rather defensive. They didn't want to believe there was a problem with where they lived. Their lives evolved around life in the city, and they seemed more concerned about the conveniences of their lifestyle than acknowledging that perhaps they needed to make a change for the well-being of their child. How many parents watch their children suffer and don't know there is better way? How many parents would make the sacrifice to leave a toxic environment for the health of the family?

It has been fascinating to watch over the years as I have made health food products, nutritional supplements, and animal care products that too often the animal care products outsell the children's vitamins and enzymes.

It isn't easy to make a big change like moving from the city to the country, but we can make our living environment cleaner and safer with the food we eat, the water we drink, and the cleaning products we use, etc. We can make our home environment as non-toxic as possible.

Families should take advantage of any opportunity to go to the country or the mountains and get away from the city. Summer is a wonderful time for camping and spending time in nature. Take away all the processed food for a couple of weeks, and it is amazing how behaviors change. That also includes the elimination of cell phones and battery-powered electronics. The idea is to get away from the modern world and all of its conveniences.

All of these things are ways to improve the quality of our lives and help us overcome different afflictions and physical problems, but what is the root cause of this gluten intolerance, celiac disease, allergies, and so many new maladies that we see today? Perhaps a look into the history of the ancient grain of einkorn with the evolution of our modern wheat will give us some answers.

ENDNOTES

1   Tersigni C, et al. Celiac disease and reproductive disorders: meta-analysis of epidemiologic associations and potential pathogenic mechanisms. *Hum Reprod Update.* 2014 Mar 11.
2   Raijput R, et al. Primary infertility as a rare presentation of celiac disease. *Fertil Steril.* 2010 Dec;94(7):2771.
3   Farthing MF, et al. Male gonadal function in coeliac disease: III. Pituitary regulation. *Clin Endocrinol. (Oxf).* 1983 Dec;19(6):661-71.
4   Stazi A, et al. Celiac disease and its endocrine and nutritional implications on male reproduction. *Minerva Med.* 2004 Jun;95(3):243-54.
5   http://www.cdc.gov/nchs/fastats/obesity-overweight.htm.
6   http://www.who.int/mediacentre/factsheets/fs311/en/.
7   Davis W, MD. *Wheat Belly,* Rodale, 2011:x.

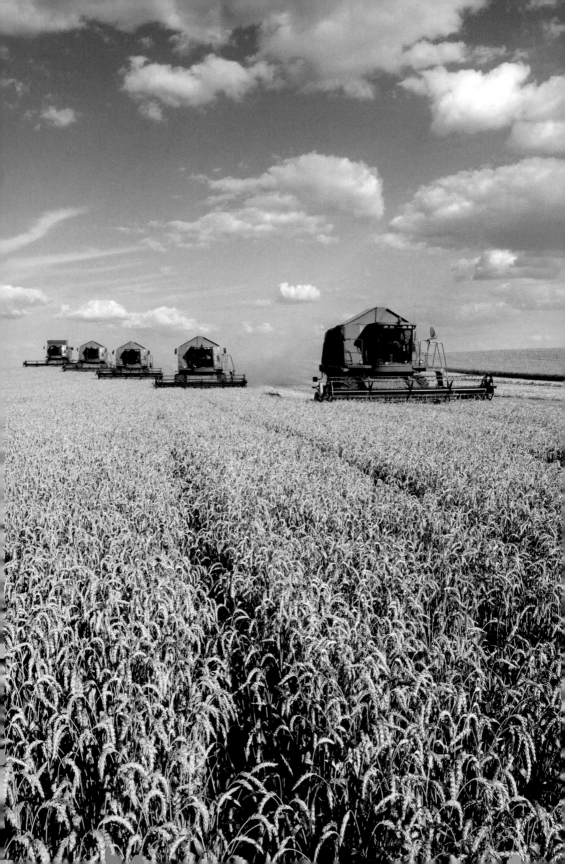

CHAPTER 3
Modern Hybrid Wheat

"The Bible says, 'Give us this day our daily bread.' Eating bread is nearly a religious commandment. But einkorn, Biblical heirloom wheat of our ancestors, is something modern humans never eat."[1]

The author of those words is Dr. Mark Hyman, a board certified, family practice physician and *New York Times* best-selling author. The modern hybrid wheat that we buy today and find in our breads, cereals, pastries, bagels, and all the various wheat products we eat, is not the wheat that gave our ancestors health. It is so far removed from God's original einkorn wheat that it could be branded the "Staff of Death and Disease."

The original einkorn grain (*Triticum monococcum*) had (and still has!) 1 genome (meaning the genetic material, DNA) and 14 chromosomes (2 sets of 7). What happened to this wheat of ancient times that was so nutritious? Why are many doctors saying that our modern hybrid wheat is so harmful?

DR. NORMAN BORLAUG AND DWARF WHEAT

How and when did wheat change so drastically?

In the mid-1900s, biologist Dr. Norman Borlaug worked on a wheat-cross-breeding project in Mexico. The intent was to create a wheat variety that would increase production yields and be resistant to a wheat fungus called rust, which was causing production losses.

Borlaug's work accomplished both tasks. He crossbred traditional wheat with a Japanese dwarf wheat that had a shorter, sturdier stalk to hold up the heavier wheat head. The new stalks were now shorter so that there was less straw in the field for the farmers to discard, making harvesting faster and more efficient.

Wheat yields doubled in Mexico and India with his new dwarf wheat. The heads were larger and yielded more kernels, so naturally, more tonnage per acre was produced than the traditional wheat produced. Dr. Davis writes, "The average yield on a modern North American farm is more than tenfold greater than farms of a century ago."[2]

Dr. Borlaug was awarded the Nobel Peace Prize, the Presidential Medal of Freedom, and the Congressional Medal of Honor, one of only seven persons to ever receive all three awards. The big flaw in Borlaug's achievement was that *no* animal or safety testing was done on this new, hybridized dwarf wheat.

MODERN HYBRIDIZATION

Hybridization is a word that might be unfamiliar to many people. It is a modern word about a modern way of combining two different seeds or plant species to engineer a new plant. It is man's way of changing Mother Nature to create something bigger and better, so they think.

The wheat of today is not the same as the wheat of ancient times. Talking about these two different wheat varieties is like comparing apples and oranges. The ancient wheat is Mother Nature's gift, and today's wheat is man's creation.

Many research papers have been written about wheat because of the huge rise in worldwide gluten intolerance and celiac disease. Many researchers and scientists are asking what is causing these problems. What has caused this intolerance and intestinal dysfunction that is being linked to autism, fibromyalgia, arthritis, diabetes, and even cancer? Is it possible that this ancient staff of life has become the staff of death and disease today?

Hybridization can take place naturally with Mother Nature like when one species is growing in a field on one side of the creek, and another species is growing in another field on the other side of the creek or even on the other side of the valley. As they start to pollinate and breezes blow, the pollen moves from one crop to the other; and as a result, we have a crossbred plant or what is called hybridization. It is a natural occurrence of Mother Nature; but when man steps in and forces the process over and over, problems develop.

Gene splicing is completely manipulated by scientists in laboratories. Modern wheat cultivars belong to two biological species. One is classified as bread wheat, *triticum aestivum*, and has 2N = 6X = 42 chromosomes, valued for the baking of high-rising bread. The other is hard durum wheat, *triticum turgidum*, which has 2N=4X=28 chromosomes and is used for pasta and low-rising bread.

Other triticum species originate from more primitive cultivars. Einkorn, *Triticum monococcum* L., is a diploid wheat, containing just 14 chromosomes.

When we review the wheat cytogenetics that was published by Reilly in 1965, Sears in 1969, Miller in 1987, and Fieldman in 1995, they were very clear that some domesticated forms of wheat have a diploid chromosome number 2N=2X=14 and contain two sets of a single genome, designated AA.

Other wheats are tetraploid, 2N=4X=28, and combine two distinct genomes, either BBAA or GGAA. Others are hexaploid, 2N=6X=42 chromosomes and contain three different genomes, BBAADD.

Domestic wheat falls into three chromosomal groups, diploid wheat, tetraploid wheat, and hexaploid wheat.

Forms within each group are interfertile and share the same chromosome constitution. In contrast, hybrids between groups are highly sterile. The taxonomic classification of domesticated wheat and their closely related wild types was written about by Van Slageren in 1994 and is based on these cytogenetic criteria.

Researchers are investigating ancient einkorn wheat as possibly being safe for celiac patients. Many people ask, "Isn't one wheat just like another?" Well, no. Dr. William Davis points out that 14-chromosome einkorn has one genome (A); emmer, with 28 chromosomes, has the A and B genomes; and 42-chromosome *Triticum aestivum,* today's hybridized wheat, has three genomes, A, B, and D. In his book he notes, "Indeed, genes located in the D genome are those most frequently pinpointed as the source of the glutens that trigger celiac disease."[3]

So scientists are seeking a different grain that is safe for celiac patients. Research on this topic is cautious, which is understandable, considering the physical pain and grief this condition causes those who ingest wheat products. Einkorn research coming from Italy has added a little hope for celiacs. A 2012 study stated that "the ancient diploid *Triticum monococcum* spp. *monococcum* wheat showed a marked reduction, even a lack of, toxicity in in vitro cellular assays, which suggested their possible use as new dietary opportunities for CD patients."[4]

Another Italian study did not draw a definite conclusion of safety of *Triticum monococcum* for celiacs but did state that *Triticum monococcum* "was, however, well tolerated by all patients providing a rationale for further investigation on the safety of this cereal for CD patients."[5]

Dwarf wheat (*Triticum aestivum*), the hybrid wheat of today, has 3 genomes and 42 chromosomes (6 sets of 7). Those extra chromosomes create new proteins that man was never meant to consume. They are foreign to the body of both man

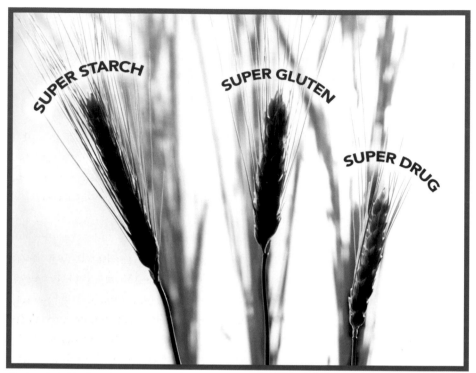

Modern hybrid wheat is a major contributor to many modern ills.

and animals and cause confusion in the digestive system.

Dr. Hyman is alarmed and has strong concerns about modern hybridized wheat and not just because of its gluten content:

> There are three major reasons that wheat, along with gluten and sugar in all their forms, is a major contributor to obesity, diabetes, heart disease, cancer, dementia, depression and so many other modern ills.

1. It contains a **Super Starch**—amylopectin A that is super fattening.
2. It contains a form of **Super Gluten** that is super-inflammatory.
3. It contains forms of a **Super Drug** that is super-addictive and makes you crave and eat more.

This is why there are now **30 percent more obese people than undernourished people in the world**, and why chronic lifestyle and dietary-driven disease kills more than twice as many people globally as infectious disease. These non-communicable, chronic diseases will cost our global economy $47 trillion over the next 20 years.[6] [Emphasis added]

In *Wheat Belly*, Dr. Davis explains that 5 percent of wheat proteins of a hybrid from two-parent species are unique, not found in either parent. Another hybridizing experiment produced **14 new proteins** not found in either parent plant. He compared century-old strains of wheat to the hybridized wheat and found that the modern versions "express a higher quantity of genes for gluten proteins that are associated with celiac disease."[7]

Dr. Davis told CBS This Morning: "There's a new protein in this thing called gliadin. It is not gluten. I am not talking about people with gluten sensitivities and celiac disease. I am talking about everyone else. This thing [gliadin] binds into the opiate receptors in your brain and in most people stimulates appetite such that we consume 440 more calories per day, 365 days per year."[8]

What will this hybrid wheat cost us in health? It has a more fattening starch, highly inflammatory gluten, and gliadin protein that continually makes us hungry for more carbohydrates. But the worst problem hybrid wheat causes, with its problematic gluten, is the damage to the digestive tract.

We need to educate ourselves and learn how we can prevent the problems that come from eating modern wheat and all the foods made from this wheat flour as well as other hybridized grains. How can we protect our families, and what are the alternatives today?

ENDNOTES

1   http://www.huffingtonpost.com/dr-mark-hyman/wheat-gluten_b_1274872.html?view=screen.
2   Davis W, MD. *Wheat Belly*, Rodale, 2011:14.
3   Ibid., 38-39.
4   Gianfrani C, et al. Immunogenicity of monococcum wheat in celiac patients. *Am J Clin Nutr.* 2012 Dec;96(6):1339-45.
5   Zanini B, et al. Search for atoxic cereals: a single blind, cross-over study on the safety of a single dose of *Triticum monococcum,* in patients with celiac disease. *BMC Gastroenterol.* 2013 May 24;13(1):92.
6   http://www.huffingtonpost.com/dr-mark-hyman/wheat-gluten_b_1274872.html?view=screen.
7   Davis, Ibid., 26.
8   http://www.cbsnews.com/news/modern-wheat-a-perfect-chronic-poison-doctor-says/.

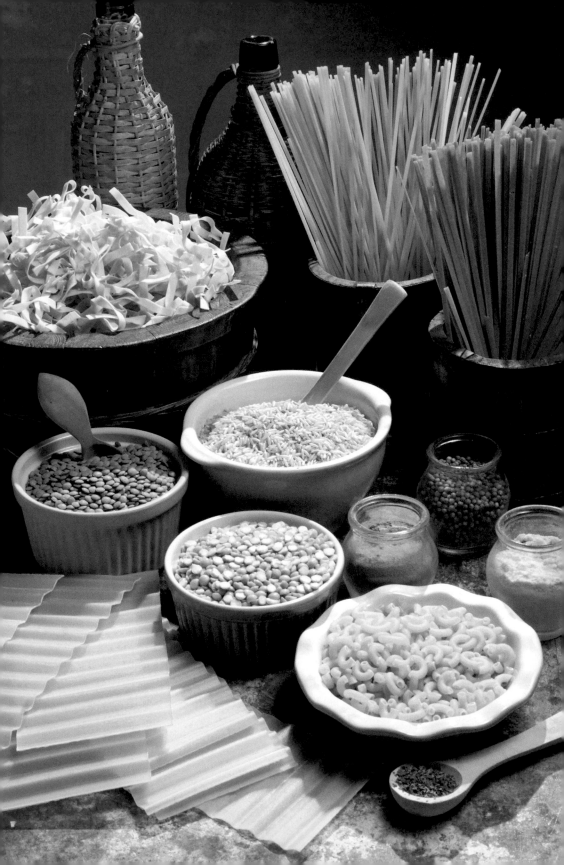

CHAPTER 4

Gluten: Friend or Foe?

An immediate and direct food allergy to wheat is rare, affecting only 0.2-0.5 percent of the population. Celiac disease is found in about 1 percent of Americans. However, the new and growing pathology is gluten sensitivity, where eating gluten causes gastrointestinal problems; and a new study estimated that 6 percent of the U.S. population suffers from this, despite no celiac or wheat allergy diagnosis.[1]

The dark side of gluten and other man-made wheat proteins has finally become a hot topic of research and debate. Wheat germ agglutinin is not only a direct intestinal toxin in animals, but it disrupts normal gastric function, according to researchers at the University of Maryland.[2]

Gluten is found in wheat and related grains in the Triticum family of grassy grains or cereal grains, which include barley, bulgur wheat, durum wheat, farro, graham, kamut, rye, semolina, spelt, triticale, and einkorn. **The only one of all of the above-mentioned grains that has not been hybridized or genetically modified today is einkorn, *Triticum monococcum*.**

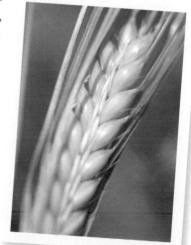

Barley

Thousands of years ago, the great evolution and natural hybridization of grains took place, and man ate them because they sustained life with a good balance of protein, minerals, fiber, and carbohydrates.

But today many people believe that our digestive system was never designed to digest processed grains and flours, and some people

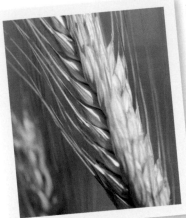

Triticale

believe that we don't have the ability to fully digest gluten molecules into their component amino acids.

I personally question this. I don't think that God would create nutritious grains, seeds, grasses, and other similar foods and not expect man to eat them; and surely He knew that through time, nature would crossbreed and make natural and nutritious variations of these foods as well.

Our teeth were built for tearing through meat and plants and grinding them, thus creating the first phase of digestion with the salivary fluids in our mouth that enter the stomach to begin that process and also to stimulate the release of hydrochloric acid and pepsin in the stomach.

However, I also don't think God expected man to create unnatural crossbreeding in a laboratory. When man began to hybridize the grains over and over, creating unnatural structures such as today's wheat, *Triticum aestivum,* with its 42 chromosomes and huge payload of unfamiliar proteins that the body cannot digest, then man created his own punishment for having messed with nature.

A physician and expert on the physiological effects of wheat, William Davis, MD, summed it up very nicely: "It is the ultimate hubris of modern humans that we can change and manipulate the genetic code of another species to suit our needs. . . . genetic modification and hybridization of the plants we call food crops remain crude science still fraught with unintended effects. . . ."[3]

Our bodies are created to digest natural wild grasses such as einkorn (with the 14 chromosomes), not the hybridized, 42-chromosome monstrosities that we don't have the proper enzymes to digest.

For those who have gluten sensitivity, a natural gluten from a 14-chromosome grass like einkorn will likely not cause a reaction because the body recognizes it as a digestible food. But when a hybridized food with an unnatural protein structure created from a 42-chromosome man-made wheat enters the gut, the body has extreme difficulty digesting and recognizing it.

Gluten is an important element in your food chain, because it is a protein and your body needs protein. However, you can obtain protein from many different types of foods and food combinations. You do not have to rely on gluten alone.

Some people think that all grain that contains gluten is toxic and bad. But that is not true because not all glutens are bad. **There are good glutens and bad glutens, and we need to know the difference.**

IS ALL GLUTEN BAD?

The gluten that comes in our modern, hybridized wheat is incompatible with the human body and is likely to contribute to autoimmune diseases, inflammation, and a host of other unintended and undesirable effects.

It has been fascinating over the last five years to see how so many gluten-free foods have come into the market. Five years ago it was almost impossible to find gluten-free foods. Two years ago they started coming into the health food stores and in special aisles of the supermarkets. Now there are many gluten-free foods to choose from in the health food sections.

There is a big difference between glutens, just like there is a big difference between grains.

We were designed to eat both grains and carnivore-type foods. God made us all different and individually unique with our personalities, chemistries, likes and dislikes, digestive functions, and body types, etc. However, He also made us with a lot of similarities between O, A, AB, and B blood types.

It shouldn't be about a fad, and we shouldn't spend our time arguing over who is right and who is wrong, because what is right for me is not necessarily right for someone else.

There are believed to be 3 million people in the United States with celiac disease and unknown numbers more who suffer from gluten sensitivity. But eating gluten-free seems to becoming a fad, and that gives me a great deal of concern. Fad diets come and go, and yet obesity and the decline of health continue. One person may lose weight by going on a gluten-free diet, but in 10 years will that person be as healthy as the first year of eating gluten-free? A gluten-free diet is a dangerous fad because we are looking at the wrong culprit.

The Right Kind of Gluten

Why is gluten—the **right kind** of gluten—important and beneficial in the diet?

Since the beginning of time, diet has been a major factor influencing gut microbiota (the trillions of beneficial microbes in the human intestine) diversity and functionality.

COMPOSITION OF GLUTEN

Gluten is a composite of several different proteins: glutenin and gliadin (in wheat), hordein (in barley), and secalin (in rye). They are elastic proteins known as prolamins.

Gliadin is alcohol soluble and glutenin is soluble only in diluted acids or alkalines. Prolamin and gluten compose about 80 percent of the protein contained in wheat seed. Being insoluble in water, it can be purified by washing away the associated starch.

These protein composites, which give gluten its unique structure and function, are the proteins responsible for triggering gluten intolerance symptoms, celiac disease symptoms, and a non-celiac gluten sensitivity.

THE PROBLEM WITH GLUTEN

So what really is the problem with gluten? When gluten from man-made 42-chromosome "engineered" wheat enters the bloodstream, it can trigger immune responses that damage the lining of the small intestine, which then interfere with the absorption of nutrients and cause symptoms that can lead to other problems such as osteoporosis, nerve damage, seizures, infertility, etc.

Prolamins are part of the polypeptide chains sometimes referred to as peptides and are found in abundance in hybridized wheat. These wreak havoc by triggering inflammatory responses in the gut and interfering with intestinal absorption of nutrients.

The gliadins are glutelins, which are insoluble in water and are altered by heat, reacting with and crosslinking with themselves and other proteins. This is how gluten causes the dough to rise when baking bread. Gluten gives bread, pasta, cake, etc., that nice fluffy, but sticky, texture and holds them together so they don't crumble or fall apart.

The gliadins have been altered through genetic manipulation and hybridization, creating novel and potentially harmful proteins in the process, which can trigger not only gluten intolerance but also a host of other health issues such as systemic inflammation, poor cognitive functioning, and impaired digestion. The glutelins have also been known to trigger damaging autoimmune (pro-inflammatory) response in people with genetic susceptibility to gluten.

Dr. William Davis says the problem with gluten is that, "The gliadin protein of wheat exerts opioid effects on the human brain that, via the tetra- and pentapeptide digestates of gliadin, stimulate calorie consumption: 400 more calories per day, every day. The effect is blocked by naloxone/naltrexone, opiate blocking drugs."[4] Dr. Davis continues:

> The gliadin protein has been known (Fasano, et al.) to increase small intestinal permeability, permitting entry of polypeptide antigens into the bloodstream/lymph, which is suspected to be the first step in generating autoimmunity. Wheat germ agglutinin, a direct intestinal toxin in animals, disrupts normal gastric function in the small intestinal and colonic mucosa. Unique forms of alpha-amylase inhibitors are suspected to be among the factors responsible for the explosive increase in childhood allergies and asthma.[5]

These changes in wheat took place because scientists thought they could create a bigger yield. They said the stalk had to be shorter to hold up the larger seed heads. The change in structure would make both the harvest and threshing time faster and more effective, besides increasing the yield. It doesn't seem that there was any concern for the changes in the genomes and chromosomes of this wheat that had been such a nutritious food that would now make this "new" wheat so toxic to the people of the world.

GLUTEN SENSITIVITY

Some scientists say that 6 percent of Americans suffer from some gluten sensitivity. Other scientists assert that gluten can lead to severe intestinal distress for those who have celiac disease, but those who don't have gluten sensitivity can eat it without any problem.

But how much man-made wheat products will be consumed before that gluten sensitivity manifests? It is only going to be a matter of time, because undigested gluten creates inflammation in the gut and in the gut lining, which produces toxins that permeate the mucosal wall, enter the bloodstream, and wreak havoc in the brain receptors, creating other food intolerances that may not even be related to gluten.

Unfortunately, once there is inflammation in the villi of the small intestine (the very tiny structures responsible for the absorption of nutrients from the digestion of food) and is left untreated, many problems develop such as diarrhea, bloating, and abdominal pain that are related to diseases such as irritable bowel syndrome, colitis, diverticulitis, and intestinal cancer, resulting from a host of nutritional deficiencies.

Today, genetically modified and hybridized wheat grows on over 1 million acres of land in just the U.S. and has taken the once-rare celiac disease statistic affecting 1 American in 10,000 to 1 in 133 today, due largely to the hybridization that caused the enrichment of the gliadin/alpha 9 gene, found in modern, hybridized wheat, which was virtually non-existent in the wheat before 1960.

These inflammatory responses have grown astronomically, to the point where celiac disease is considered one of the most common genetic disorders in the Western world by the Center for Celiac Disease Research at the University of Maryland, according to a 2003 study published in the Archives of Internal Medicine. "Celiac disease appears to be a more common but neglected disorder than has generally been recognized in the United States."[6]

Some people argue that hybridized wheat is essential for its B vitamins and fiber, not taking into consideration that there are other sources of B vitamins and fiber. However, we certainly do not have to continue to hybridize, genetically modify, and enrich our food with indigestible synthetic additives.

GLUTEN INTOLERANCE

Gluten intolerance has been implicated with rampant depression, anxiety, and hyperactivity in the United States. The number of young children who are suffering from depression, anxiety, and are taking drugs to calm down their hyperactivity is astounding.

These drugs used to treat these cognitive disorders are chemicals that poison the body and should always be avoided. It is appalling how many teachers think an energetic child naturally has ADHD (Attention Deficit/Hyperactivity Disorder) and should be put on drugs.

These kinds of drugs shut down the creative ability to think and dream. The moment a child is put on a drug to depress or "quiet" the mind, you have put the child in a box, closed the lid, and locked it possibly for life.

Similarly, any individual who suffers with depression or anxiety should first ask questions like the following: "What am I eating that might not be good for me? What do I eat daily or weekly?" Then start a process of elimination.

Do we keep searching for an answer, or do we just continue as before and keep wondering what is wrong? Visiting the doctor will probably result in a prescription for a corticosteroid or an anti-inflammatory. Then when your condition gets worse and your blood pressure goes up, you will probably be told to get a prescription for a medication to lower your blood pressure. Then when you feel depressed, the doctor will likely prescribe an antidepressant. A few weeks later, when you feel a lot of anxiety, you will likely be told to get an anti-anxiety medication. You can't get off the merry-go-round, and all along it is just because you are eating hybridized wheat.

The best first step is to eliminate hybrid (dwarf) wheat and man-made wheat products from your diet. This means modern wheat and its flour. Unfortunately, man-made gluten is everywhere and embedded in thousands of commonly consumed food products; this will be extremely challenging, since 99 percent of all wheat grown in the world originates from sterile, genetically spliced-and-diced seeds.[7]

The next step would be to eliminate other gluten-containing products, including such things as lipstick and other beauty and skin-care products that might be using gluten as a binder. Search on the Internet and look for lists of household products and foods that use gluten for binding and creating a creamy texture and then avoid them.

Gluten makes dough elastic and gives it the strength and structure so that it can rise two or three times its size. It gives bread a soft, chewy texture once it is baked. It is very difficult to bake bread or a piecrust with gluten-free flour like dhokla flour made from lentils, rice flour, tapioca flour, or potato starch flour. When you take it out of the pan and try to cut it, it just falls apart. You definitely won't be making sandwiches for school with that kind of bread.

THE GLUTEN LINK

Is there a link between gluten consumption, gluten intolerance, celiac disease, and autism? Many people will argue the issue and say that gluten has nothing to do with these diseases, that they are completely unrelated. For many years parents have experimented with gluten-free diets for children with autism; and not all showed improvement in behavior, mood, or communication. Researchers found no correlation between autism and celiac disease.

However, autism and gluten intolerance may be indirectly related. Children who have symptoms of autism already have compromised digestive conditions that inhibit the assimilation of amino acids and nutrients that are essential to maintaining proper brain function, mood control, and activity response.

We cannot blame wheat gluten for the rapid increase of autism, but it is probably a contributing factor. Did the child's mother consume a lot of man-made wheat and gluten products while she was pregnant, thus contributing to the problem? Did the grandmother live on wheat throughout her life? Most likely. Did generations of mothers consuming wheat in their diet and absorbing gluten through their skin with various beauty products create a blueprinting on the DNA that was passed down through the generations, leading to an inherent weakness of gluten intolerance? That is certainly a possibility.

"Quack" Diseases Become Real

Candida and hypoglycemia were the new diseases of the 1950s and '60s that were hailed by the medical profession as "quack" diseases made up by "quack" practitioners, naturopaths, chiropractors, and homeopaths. Interestingly enough, today the medical profession and pharmaceutical companies have "claimed" those diseases as their own and concocted new drugs to treat them. As soon as there was a money-making potential, America's medical and pharmaceutical establishments embraced them full throttle.

In the 1940s, with the mechanization of harvesting, things started to change. The hybridization of wheat and the application of chemicals on our food crops became common. The chemical manufacturers were busily creating herbicides to combat weeds and grasses to give the farmers better yields and lengthen growing cycles. Scientists were in the laboratory engaged in hybridizing different crops.

Candida and hypoglycemia were unaccepted maladies in the 1950s and '60s. In 1970 fibromyalgia was not a disease. In 1980 the Epstein Barr virus was not a disease. In 1985 leaky gut syndrome was another "quack" disease that was not recognized by medical practitioners.

But what about autism, ADHD, Asperger's, depression, Parkinson's, dementia, Alzheimer's, and others? What about "brain fog" (a reduced ability to think and reason, usually caused by candida and toxins leaching from the gut into the bloodstream)? What about neurological disorders that didn't exist 75 years ago? Why do we have them today? Where will we be 10 years from now? How many children are suffering today, and where will they be 25 to 35 years from now? Even 40 to 50 years from now? Will they have children who will be born genetically aligned with these autistic behaviors that will be passed down genetically from parent to child?

It is fascinating to think of nutrition and digestion, from chewing, digesting, assimilating, and getting rid of the waste. The body is a highly complex organism that needs to function at an optimal level to perform all the necessary metabolic exchanges necessary for a healthy and vibrant life. We must do our best and always be learning and asking questions to help fight and stop the proliferation of new diseases.

We must always be thinking of the consequences of our actions. Awareness is a great beginning for solving problems and finding better ways to eat and take care of our bodies. It is ultimately our responsibility to take care of ourselves and our children. With good information and solutions for improving, we can live happy, healthy lives with energy and mental alertness.

GLUTEN-FREE DIETS

Gluten-free diets are promoted relentlessly by Hollywood, health food and nutrition stores, health advocates, and fitness buffs. Other people have jumped on the bandwagon; and the next thing you know, companies are packing aisles full of products touting their lack of stretchy wheat proteins. But for a lot of people, the gluten-free lifestyle is showing now to do more harm than good.

How can that be? For people with celiac disease, gluten is a nutritional threat, and cutting out gluten for these people is a lifesaver. Marlisa Brown, RD, author of *Gluten-Free, Hassle Free,* said, "If you skip the gluten-free goodies and focus on fruits, vegetables, lean protein, dairy, and gluten free grains like amaranth and quinoa, this can be a very healthy way of eating."[8]

Are gluten-free diets the answer? Should I eliminate all of these products?

The problem with going gluten-free is that we end up buying products loaded with sugar and other additives, which can be even worse for health. Shelly Case, R.D., author of *Gluten-Free Diet,* said, "Without gluten to bind food together, food manufacturers often use more fat and sugar to make the product more palatable."[9]

People claim that eating a gluten-free diet has changed their lives; their arthritic symptoms disappeared, their diabetic conditions disappeared, and even people with dementia have experienced improvement.

We can take anecdotal evidence and say that it shows that a gluten-free diet reduces the symptoms of many modern-day diseases. If you are a victim of one of these, to whom are you going to listen? The scientists? Or hundreds of people who testify that when they eliminated gluten, their lives were changed for the better? Most people are likely to go with the anecdotal evidence.

But what is important is that after we look at the evidence, study the science, and listen to other people, we make our own decision about what we feel is right for us, not what everyone else thinks is right for us. Experiment and if something works, then do it, irrespective of what science tells you; and if it continues to work, then it must be right for you.

The wrong gluten-free diet can lead to other problems that in time could become a major issue. For example, if a woman 20 to 40 years of age adheres to a gluten-free diet, it could take five years before other problems start to manifest. At 50 to 60 years of age, she is likely to see a greater symptom of low estrogen and the risk of greater osteoporosis-type symptoms.

A young woman in her 20s or 30s who goes on a gluten-free diet will likely have low estrogen and problems conceiving and carrying to full term due to a folate deficiency. Folate is very critical for a woman menstruating and who is going to carry a child to full term.

People on gluten-free diets for 10 years will likely see an entire host of symptoms that will originate out of the nutritional deficiencies. Sometimes eliminating something from your diet creates an imbalance someplace else. We need to be careful to not get caught up in the fad-food diet and the "gluten-is-bad" revolution.

Dr. Daniel A. Leffler, assistant professor of medicine at Harvard University and director of clinical research at the Celiac Center at Beth Israel Deaconess Medical Center in Boston, states, "People who are sensitive to gluten may feel better, but a larger portion will derive no significant benefit from the practice. They'll simply waste their money, because these products are expensive."[10] They are also loaded with sugar and additives.

Over 3 million people in the U.S. who have been diagnosed with celiac disease have to follow a strict gluten-free diet, since even small amounts of gluten will trigger debilitating gastrointestinal discomfort, with extreme cramping, pain, severe bloating, and diarrhea, followed by headaches, even hallucinations, and the loss of consciousness in extreme conditions.

Interestingly, Peter H. R. Green, MD, the director of the Celiac Disease Center at Columbia University, states, "The market for gluten-free products is exploding. Why exactly we don't know. Many people may just perceive that a gluten-free diet is healthier."[11]

A healthier diet would cure many ills, but the fat- and sugar-laden gluten-free products are not healthy. People are eating more processed food than at any time in history; they are eating more sugar than ever before; and they are eating foods with more additives, colorings, food preservatives, and stabilizers. They are eating more foods sprayed with chemicals and synthetic fertilizers; and crops are now grown in ground that has been sprayed with glyphosates in popular pesticides and other chemicals.

To bring about balance in the dietary intake of the people in our world today, we should not eliminate one thing that is essential to the body to prevent something that was caused by a nutritional deficiency in the beginning, which was primarily from enzyme and mineral deficiency.

Back in the 1980's, a book was written called *The Yeast Connection*. In that book Dr. William G. Crook said to eliminate all yeast from your diet.[12] That is like saying that if your tires bump when you go down the road, take them off and drive your car without tires or that you want to run in the Kentucky Derby but forgot your bridle and saddle.

Yeast is loaded with B vitamins, which support and sustain pancreatic functions and proper glucose/insulin ratios. Yeast is not your problem. Indigestion and the fermentation of the yeast are your problems. The foods you put into your diet, like sugar, combine with yeast and create fermentation. Yeast without sugar will not ferment. It is like comparing yeast that you put on a sterile plate with yeast that you mix with sugar. Yeast grows in the presence of sugar; so if we eat too much sugar, we have fermentation when we eat foods containing yeast—and that is the problem.

Using essential oils sometimes causes a rash because you don't have proper digestion or the body is toxic. Over the years, you may have developed a phenolic allergy because you are sulphur deficient because you weren't eating foods that supplied the sulphur you needed, or you weren't taking a mineral supplement. With a sulphur deficiency, you may experience an allergic reaction to food like asparagus, broccoli, and cauliflower or to the phenols in essential oils.

It is not the cabbage, the broccoli, or the essential oils that are the problem. It is a metabolic imbalance and dysfunction in your body.

Why do we get rashes? People get psoriasis and eczema because of a toxic overload in their body, and the liver and spleen cannot filter the pathogens, the inorganic, or organic matter that have not been digested or broken down for elimination. If the bucket is full, one drop will make it spill over. A rash is just the spillover from having a toxic body tell you, "I need help; empty my bucket." That bucket would be very good for people to check every six months.

Essential oils rich in d-limonene represent the safest and most effective way to naturally cleanse the liver and increase glutathione. Researchers at the St. Radbound University Hospital in the Netherlands found that one of the most powerful ways to improve liver detoxification and increase glutathione are limonene-rich nutrients such as orange and lemon oils.[13]

A study at the University of Minnesota found that limonene was able to counter the liver-damaging effects of paracetamol by enhancing detoxification enzymes. "Dietary D-limonene (1.0% diet for 10 days) maintained liver GSH concentrations at 92% of control values in the paracetamol-challenged mouse."[14] Only 1% of their diet with added limonene was enough to almost completely counter drug-induced liver damage.

Orange oil, which is rich in d-limonene, can also protect the stomach from damage from gluten and other man-made wheat proteins. According to researchers at Sao Paolo State University in Brazil, orange oil represents "a promising target for the development of a new drug for the prevention of gastric damage."[15]

If we use natural and wild-crafted essential oils, eat organic food, read the labels, and avoid what we know is not good for us, we have a better chance of being free of those things that might make us sick or contaminate our body.

THE ENZYME CONNECTION

Eating foods devoid of enzymes naturally creates an enzyme deficiency. I haven't yet seen an enzyme therapy used for gluten intolerance or celiac disease, except for what I did in my clinic years ago. One person had celiac disease that caused diverticulitis, and another person had celiac disease resulting in Crohn's disease. Both of these people first focused on cleansing their body. Both of them had an excess of candida. Every person in my clinic who had a gluten intolerance and celiac disease had candida overgrowth issues and were also hypoglycemic. A couple of people had early onset diabetes Type 2; and some celiac sufferers had arthritis, fibromyalgia, and even both.

Celiac disease is described as an autonomic nervous system (ANS) disorder, where the immune system attacks itself. Why would the body attack itself? Why would the body see gluten as an invader to fight?

When a baby is born, it has several hundreds of enzymes; but many are at low levels, which is why babies are given only liquids to drink in the beginning. Enzymes can take five to ten months to develop to optimal levels, which is the reason that we generally start with soft, simple foods around four to six months to see how well the baby does with its digestion.

Amylase is sometimes absent or very low at birth but is expected to be fortified through nursing. Amylase helps in the digestion of starches and is necessary to break down simple sugars and carbohydrates. If the infant is not nursed or has insufficient pancreatic secretion of amylase, then raw goat milk, similar to mother's milk, is a good way for the baby to get added amylase. If there isn't sufficient amylase, then the baby may have problems with digestion that may be detected by excessive gas, crying because of stomach pains, throwing up, restless sleep, and an unhappy disposition.

Undigested food causes fermentation, generating toxins that separate the tight junctions in the villi tract, releasing gastric molecules into the bloodstream that lead to exaggerated allergic conditions and create inflammation in the gastrointestinal lining.

Infants who are not nursed are usually given baby formula, and that inhibits the natural cultivar of acidophilus lactobacillus bifidus, which is critical for the absorption of proteins. If the proteins are not digested, they comingle with the fermentation of sugars, carbohydrates, and glucoses and feed the *Candida albicans* in the gut that goes into an overgrowth cycle.

Once candida goes into the overgrowth cycle, it attaches anywhere along the lining of the gut and grows roots just like a tree; and those roots create porosities (holes) in the gastric lining that allow undigested food and toxins to enter the bloodstream.

This cycle is exacerbated if the liver is toxic. Drugs, prescription drugs, POPs (persistent organic pollutants), chemicals, and PCBs (polychlorinated biphenyls) can all stress the liver, damage the neurons, and add to the problem of undigested food.

Certain molecules from various essential oils such as Balsam Fir, Ledum, Frankincense, Palo Santo, Ocotea, Dorado Azul, Helichrysum, and citrus oils like Lemon, Orange, Spearmint, and Peppermint have chelating properties that are able to penetrate the blood-brain barrier and help counter the toxic overload.

Gut microbiota, gluten-free diets, celiac disease, immunity, probiotics, prebiotics, and polysaccharides are all fundamental issues that should be studied more.

A year ago I was eating good 7-grain and 9-grain organic breads. Yet the more I ate, the more my old broken bones and joints started to ache and become inflamed, even to the point that I became concerned that maybe I was developing bone cancer, simply because I have lost several family members to cancer over the past 30 years. So I decided to have a checkup and a bone scan to know exactly what was going on in my body. Thankfully, the tests were all negative, so I decided to go on a gluten-free diet and immediately felt better.

If the "Service Engine" light comes on in the dashboard of your car, you will either pull out the service manual to find out why the red light came on, or you will take your car to the mechanic and ask why the light came on. The mechanic will look at it and tell you what the problem is so that you can take care of it.

When you feel something unusual or uncomfortable developing in your body, go to a physician and get a diagnosis. Use the physician's ability and knowledge to give you information, so you can make correct choices about how to care for yourself.

Doctors are not nutritionists and usually don't believe in natural medicine. They are primarily trained to diagnose and treat through drug intervention and/or surgery. They are not trained to heal the body naturally or how to prevent disease.

We need to take responsibility for our own health and choose our path of healing. There are many natural medicine doctors, dieticians, nutritionists, acupuncturists, chiropractors, herbal therapists, and a myriad of health care professionals who study nutrition and can help you make an informed decision.

IMMUNE RESPONSE

An individual who strictly follows a gluten-free diet will naturally feel a lessening of some symptoms. Unfortunately, nutritional deficiencies and health complications are also frequently found in those individuals, and the microbiota (friendly bacteria in the intestines) of individuals following gluten-free diets will not be completely restored compared to healthy individuals.

A study conducted in Valencia, Spain, tried to determine if a gluten-free diet could lead to changes in the composition and immune properties of the gut mitochondria. Ten healthy subjects about 30 years old followed a gluten-free diet for one month, replacing the gluten-containing foods they usually ate with certified gluten-free foods with no more than 20 parts per million of gluten.

Analyses of both the fecal microbiota and dietary intakes showed that the populations of healthy bacteria (*Bifidobacterium*, *B. longum,* and *Lactobacillus*) decreased, while the potentially unhealthy bacteria increased. This led the researchers to the conclusion that the "composition of the gut microbes is susceptible to the influence of the diet, and especially, to the quality and quantity of ingested carbohydrates."[16]

This study explains that the genome of the healthy bacteria *B. longum* shows that more than 8 percent of its genes are involved in carbohydrate and polysaccharide metabolism. This could explain why the healthy bacteria were reduced. The study reported, "It also seems feasible that when the growth of beneficial bacteria is not supported due to a reduced supply of their main energy sources other bacterial groups, which can be opportunistic pathogens, can [overgrow] leading to intestinal dysbiosis."[17]

It is very interesting that the genome of these good bacteria encode many enzymes that specialize in the utilization of non-digestible carbohydrates. The change in microbial diversity seems to happen because of the reduction in polysaccharide associated with a gluten-free diet. This could explain the changes in the microbiota.

The dietary intake of these compounds usually reaches the distal portion of the colon partially undigested and therefore constitutes one of the main energy sources for the gut microbiota. It seems that these healthy bacteria *need* the carbohydrates of gluten, so it seems time to give them the GOOD gluten!

BECOME A LABEL READER

It is critical to know what you are buying. You must read the ingredients on the label. For example, you go in the grocery store to buy bread and think, "I'm not going to buy wheat bread; I'm going to buy oat bread." So you buy honey-oat grain or oatnut bread or various combinations because there is very little gluten in oats. But if you don't look at the ingredients listed on the back of the package, you are not going to know what is in it. When you do, you are going to be shocked to read that in that honey-oat bread, oats are way down on the ingredient deck; and you will notice that the three primary ingredients on the deck are wheat. The deception in our food industry revolves around marketing, and they are the best.

Here is an example of the ingredient list on a certain brand of oatnut whole grain bread:

Whole White Wheat Flour, Enriched Unbleached Wheat Flour, Malted Barley Flour, Reduced Iron, Niacin (Vitamin B3), Thiamin Mononitrate (Vitamin B1), [Thiamin (Vitamin B1)], Riboflavin (Vitamin B2), [Riboflavin (Vitamin B2)], Folic Acid (Vitamin B9)), Water, Sugar, Oat(s), Yeast, Wheat Gluten. . . .[18]

Including the ingredients that are listed as being in the "Wheat Flour Enriched Unbleached," 12 ingredients are listed before "Oat(s)."

What would be the percentage of oats in ratio to the white wheat and unbleached, enriched wheat flour, which are the two leading ingredients in that bread? Then, after oats comes the yeast, and after yeast comes wheat gluten. The oats are probably added to reduce the gluten content, but then gluten is added back into the ingredients. Does that make buying oatnut bread with low gluten a good choice?

The marketing is clever and gluten intolerant people are deceived in their efforts to do better. Be a label reader and become aware of the deception present in the food industry.

Products that are labeled "gluten free" catch the eye, and you might think that is just what you want. But read the label. You might be surprised to find that the product is full of sugar—even organic sugar, which is still just sugar—preservatives, food coloring, and all kinds of poisonous ingredients. Always read the label.

Be careful of the term "sugar free." Sugar might actually be better than the sweetener they use if it is artificial. Stay away from all artificial sweeteners. They are pure poison. Do your research. There is plenty of information on the Internet, in books, and in other written material. Many products today are using agave, stevia, cane sugar, molasses, perhaps yacon, and even fruit juices, which are all better choices.

Watch out for man-made wheat gluten, which could be hiding in the most unsuspected products. This hybrid gluten is found in traditional breads, cereals, pasta, soy sauce, ice cream, ketchup, and even beer; so all you beer drinkers are loading up on gluten. Also watch out for gluten in lipsticks, MSG, toothpaste, medications, and natural flavorings. Gluten has become a major ingredient in our diet and in many other products.

A recent research study tied glyphosate, the active ingredient found in popular weed killers and sprayed on most commercial wheat crops, to the rise of gluten intolerance, celiac disease, irritable bowel syndrome, depression, thyroid disease, kidney failure, and cancer.[19]

Another new study has shown that women whose diets include soft drinks, fatty red meat, and refined grains (pasta, crackers, and chips) have a 29-41 percent higher rate of depression than those who eat a healthier diet. Researchers at the Harvard School of Public Health followed more than 43,000 women for 12 years to document this diet-related rise in depression. The women who ate these foods also had higher levels of three biomarkers of inflammation.[20]

When the gut lining is damaged, assimilation of nutrients is greatly inhibited. Damaged villi cannot properly process and assimilate nutrients such as vitamins B3, B6, B12, and folate. Deficiencies in iron, vitamins D and K, and calcium contribute to both mental and physical impairment, causing a deficit in social interaction, communication, behavior patterns, interests, or activities that impair normal cognitive and developmental functions daily from early childhood.

Hybrid gluten is the root cause of significant digestive inflammation in a good part of society, and few folks realize this. "Gluten causes gut inflammation in at least 80% of the population and another 30% of the population develops antibodies against gluten proteins in the gut. Furthermore, 99% of the population has the genetic potential to develop antibodies against gluten."[21]

Some people say that there is no substantial evidence and that the studies are only anecdotal. Who is behind these negative statements? Where do they get their research money, grant money, or the little subsidy found in their pockets? Big pharma? Who benefits from keeping the public in the dark? Who benefits from hiding the truth? That question could be asked in many areas of life!

It is the same as the sugar companies not wanting the public to know that sugar causes cancer, heart disease, and diabetes; every disease known to man can be linked to sugar.

Gluten and sugar cause inflammation, depression, and anxiety. Gluten in hybrid wheat also causes depression and anxiety.

Warning. As the gluten-free food fad emerges into our world, more and more gluten-free products are being manufactured. This does not mean they are safe. Again, become a label reader. Most gluten-free foods are replaced with rice and corn starches. Dr. William Davis writes that "Foods made with cornstarch, rice starch, potato starch, and tapioca starch are among the few foods that increase blood sugar even *more* than wheat products."[22] Beware. These products will also contain sugar, inflammatory oils, additives, preservatives, and other unnatural ingredients that can cause depression and anxiety.

We become conditioned by the things we read and hear, and we want to believe that those who are telling us know what they are talking about. I have traveled around the world for 30 years to see things for myself. However, many articles and books are written by people who have copied someone else's information and have never seen or had the experience themselves. For example, books about frankincense have been written by people who have copied someone else's material, have never been to where the frankincense trees grow, and don't know one species from another.

With all of these gluten-related problems, it is imperative to learn about einkorn, lentil flours, and other types of legume flours that do not spike blood sugar, impair intestinal function, and cause neurological and inflammatory problems. These "ancient" and "unmodernized" flours are indeed safer and easier to ingest and much more nutritious.

THE BOTTOM LINE

So what is the bottom line that we see through all of the research that has been conducted concerning the disadvantages of a gluten-free diet and the decrease in immune response because there isn't enough gluten for gut mucosal immunity?

Although research is preliminary and has not been very extensive, there has been enough to indicate that a gluten-free diet is not the recommended way to go, except in the case of celiac disease.

Certain *types* of gluten are bad for you, but not *all* types. When the study[23] showed that increasing enterobacterial counts, bacteroides, and *E. coli* were detected in healthy adults on a gluten-free diet, there were indications that the harmful bacteria increased because the healthy bacteria were not getting nutrients from a healthy gluten, allowing the harmful bacteria to multiply freely.

The findings also suggest that patients on a gluten-free diet could be helped with dietary and nutritional counseling because they have a greater need for increasing their intake of polysaccharide and pre- and probiotics. It is most important that enzymes be taken with the pre-and probiotic and polysaccharide along with a very specific liver cleansing program.

Every celiac and gluten intolerant person should go on a very rigorous liver and gall bladder cleansing with a thyroid-supporting program that includes enzymes and good pre-and probiotic bacteria.

THE EINKORN SOLUTION

The comparison of the gluten content in different flours tells the story. Einkorn, with its 1 genome, 14 chromosomes, low glycemic index, and very low gluten levels, is definitely our best choice. It is an ancient mineral-and vitamin-dense grain that is very different from the 42-chromosome, man-made, genetically manipulated modern wheat that threatens the health of the people of the world today.

Percent Gluten Content of Flours

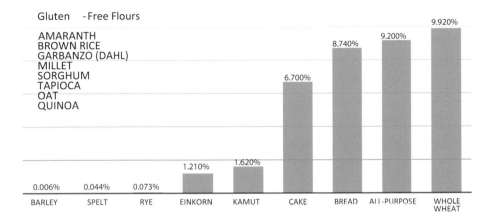

Gluten   -Free Flours

AMARANTH
BROWN RICE
GARBANZO (DAHL)
MILLET
SORGHUM
TAPIOCA
OAT
QUINOA

9.920%
9.200%
8.740%
6.700%
1.620%
1.210%
0.006%   0.044%   0.073%

BARLEY   SPELT   RYE   EINKORN   KAMUT   CAKE   BREAD   ALL-PURPOSE   WHOLE WHEAT

Gluten Content of Flours in Parts Per Million (PPM)

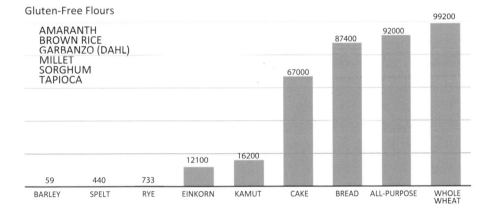

Gluten-Free Flours

AMARANTH
BROWN RICE
GARBANZO (DAHL)
MILLET
SORGHUM
TAPIOCA

99200
92000
87400
67000
16200
12100
59   440   733

BARLEY   SPELT   RYE   EINKORN   KAMUT   CAKE   BREAD   ALL-PURPOSE   WHOLE WHEAT

Special interests are pushing hard to get GMO foods accepted by the USDA and the FDA, even though mounting evidence indicates that these foods may contribute to cancer.

We need to speak up and demand that this adulteration of our food stop. Whole grain einkorn is 2½ times richer in protein than our commercial wheat, is three times higher as an antioxidant, tastes delicious, and is easily digested. Einkorn gluten does not create fermentation and permeability in the mucosal lining of the gut and is very healing and soothing to the gut lining. It is an extremely nutritious alternative to the detrimental effects of modern wheat.

My family has been eating einkorn for over a year, usually three to four times a week in pancakes, baked breads, and spaghetti. We make carrot cake and cookies that are delicious, and we continue to experiment. It is a most tasty and delicious flour; and we like combining it with quinoa, coconut, and almond flour. We make different combinations weekly for our pancakes. Einkorn combined with quinoa, amaranth, and even brown rice makes a very good balanced and sustainable food, even for gluten intolerant people. **Remember—not all glutens are created equal.**

YOU GET WHAT YOU ASK FOR

The people in the world get what they ask for. They demand cheaper prices, so they get a cheaper product. They demand something produced faster, so they get a faster process that reduces the value and the quality of what they are putting in their body. That, of course, is what has brought forth the era of fast-food diets and fast-food restaurants that are causing such a frightening increase in disease. Regarding wheat, Dr. Davis sums it up very clearly:

> In the 10,000 year journey from innocent, low-yield, not-so-baking-friendly einkorn grass to high-yield, created-in-a-laboratory, unable-to-survive-in-the-wild, suited-to-modern-tastes dwarf wheat, we've witnessed a human engineering transformation that is no different from pumping livestock with antibiotics and hormones, while confining them to a factory warehouse. Perhaps we can recover from this catastrophe called agriculture, but a big first step is to recognize what we've done to this thing called "wheat."[24]

I believe it is time for us to roll back the clock and return to our ancestral "staff of life" before geneticists begin tinkering and manipulating plant DNA to create profit-friendly synthetic wheat and flour. This is why ancient einkorn, the aboriginal food of civilization with a pure unmodified DNA will determine our future.

ENDNOTES

1   Gil-Humanes J, et al. Reduced-gliadin wheat bread: an alternative to the gluten-free diet for consumers suffering gluten-related pathologies. *PLoS One.* 2014 Mar 12;9(3):e90898.
2   Fasano A, de Magistris L. Antibodies against food antigens in patients with autistic spectrum disorders. *Biomed Res Int.* 2013;2013:729349.
3   Davis W, MD. *Wheat Belly,* Rodale, 2011:228.

4   Davis W, MD. http://www.wheatbellyblog.com/2013/03/give-harvard-health-a-piece-of-your-mind/comment-page-1/.

5   Ibid.

6   Davis, page 24.

7   http://www.womenshealthmag.com/health/gluten-free-diet.

8   Ibid.

9   http://www.womenshealthmag.com/health/gluten-free-diet.

10   http://www.health.harvard.edu/blog/going-gluten-free-just-because-heres-what-you-need-to-know-201302205916.

11   http://www.webmd.com/diet/healthy-kitchen-11/truth-about-gluten.

12   Crook WG. *The Yeast Connection.* Vancouver, Washington: Vintage Books, 1989.

13   van Lieshout EM, Posner GH, Woodard BT, Peters WH. Effects of the sulforaphane analog compound 30, indole-3-carbinol, D-limonene or relafen on glutathione S-transferases and glutathione peroxidase of the rat digestive tract. *Biochim Biophys Acta.* 1998 Mar 2;1379(3):325-36.

14   Reicks MM, Crankshaw D. Effects of D-limonene on hepatic microsomal monooxygenase activity and paracetamol-induced glutathione depletion in mouse. *Xenobiotica.* 1993 Jul;23(7):809-19.

15   Moraes TM, et al. Effects of limonene and essential oil from Citrus aurantium on gastric mucosa: role of prostaglandins and gastric mucus secretion. *Chem Biol Interact.* 2009 Aug 14;180(3):499-505.

16   Sanz Y. Effects of a gluten-free diet on gut microbiota and immune function in healthy adult humans. *Gut Microbes.* 2010 May-Jun;1(3):135-7.

17   Ibid.

18   Foodfacts.com. Oroweat Oatnut Whole Grain Sliced Bread (18 Slices). http://www.foodfacts.com/ci/nutritionfacts/whole-grain/oroweat-oatnut-whole-grain-sliced-bread-18-slices/83493.

19   Samsel A, Seneff S. Glyphosate, pathways to modern diseases II: Celia sprue and gluten intolerance. *Interdiscip Toxicol.* 2013 Dec;6(4):159-184.

20   Lucas M, et al. Inflammatory dietary pattern and risk of depression among women. *Brain Behav Immun.* 2014 Feb;36:46-53.

21   McCarthy. Gluten Free. Neurometabolic Solutions. http://greenvillehealth.com/gluten-free.

22   Davis, p. 72.

23   Sanz Y. Op cited.

24   Davis, p. 228.

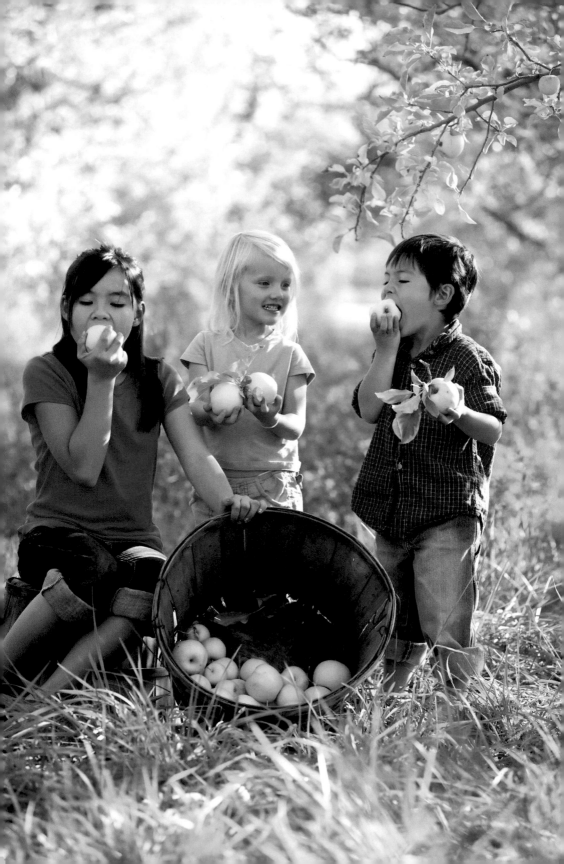

CHAPTER 5

Enzymes

Enzyme deficiencies are a growing problem every day and, I believe, are another cause of gluten intolerance and celiac disease.

WHAT ARE ENZYMES?

What are enzymes? Are they important? What do they do?

Enzymes are proteins produced by living organisms. The same variety of amino acids that occur in all living things make up enzymes. Why do these proteins act differently in the body? Because they are catalysts that create many essential biochemical reactions and changes that are essential for consumption or altering in the daily functional chemical metabolic processes of the body, they facilitate chemical reactions in the body very quickly. Without enzymes, some metabolic processes would happen very slowly or not at all.

Enzymes are found in every living cell in plants, animals, and the human body. Ancient people believed plants were magical as they watched them grow and change colors. They learned that aging meat gave it a better flavor and made it more tender and easier to digest. Little was known that the enzymatic activity was breaking down the food process and starting the decaying process. For example, sauerkraut is made by a process called lacto-fermentation. To put it (fairly) simply: A beneficial bacteria is present on the surface of the cabbage and, in fact, all fruits and vegetables. Lactobacillus is the same bacteria that is found in yogurt and many other cultured products. When submerged in a brine (water highly saturated with salt), the bacteria begin to convert sugars in the cabbage into lactic acid; this is a natural preservative that inhibits the growth of harmful bacteria.

Without enzymes, plants and grass would not grow, seeds would not germinate, flowers would not bloom, tomatoes would not turn red, and bananas would not turn yellow as they ripen. It also takes enzymes to convert sugars in a plant to essential oils. Enzymes are involved in every process, like digesting, breathing, and even thinking.

Enzymes are food potentiators. They make food available and enhance absorption and utilization of nutrients.

For example, the enzyme phytase is extremely valuable in helping to make many important minerals digestible and able to improve human health. Magnesium, calcium, and zinc are mostly biologically unavailable in many fruits and vegetables, so only a fraction of these are actually absorbed without the help of enzymes. Absorption studies show that phytase significantly increases iron and zinc bioavailability from phytate-rich foods.[1,2]

Enzyme production decreases in the absence of living food and with disease, stress, and petrochemicals. Inhibitors of enzyme production are any substance that is made of a petrochemical such as aspirin, acetaminophen, ibuprofen, antibiotics, cleaning solvents, household cleaners, microwave radiation, and heat over 120 degrees.

Our bodies were created with over 3,000 different kinds of enzymes, all with their own job description. We should have millions of enzymes when we are living in a healthy state. When our enzyme reserves start to diminish, we become bipolar, catch a cold or the flu, get arthritis, or have allergies, autism, Parkinson's, inflammation, cancer, digestive problems, heart disease, hormone deficiencies, strokes, and even gluten intolerance, celiac disease, and headaches.

Enzymes are a large part of the answer to all of these various conditions, regardless of whether it is Parkinson's, rheumatoid arthritis, or cancer.

The three primary classifications of enzymes are digestive enzymes, food enzymes, and metabolic enzymes.

When enzymes are disrupted, they lose their ability to function. Each enzyme has a specific blueprint and function. Biochemical functions in the body require enzymes, which facilitate the building of compounds, from the body's raw materials, to transporting elements throughout the body, breaking down substances such as food, and eliminating toxins and chemical wastes.

Enzymes are naturally occurring chemical compounds that orchestrate other chemical functions. Foods are made up of chemical elements that require enzymes to break them down and prepare them to be used by the body. Enzymes unlock a host of nutrients and liberate minerals, vitamins, and proteins to be engaged in body functions. They play a major role in every metabolic process in the body, from glandular function and support to hormone production and toxic waste disposal. Enzymes facilitate digestion and assimilation and also amplify the effect of hormones.

Enzymes are in all food products. Supplemental enzymes come from plant, microbial, and animal sources. Plant and microbial sources have a wider range, although not every enzyme has equal potential or all ranges in all people.

Food enzymes start in the mouth. Ptyalin, which is found only in saliva, immediately begins to break down starches and unlock vitamins even before they arrive at the fundus (the greater curvature) of the stomach for digestion. Some people consider ptyalin the most efficient enzyme, especially for starch digestion. The longer you chew your food, the more ptyalin is released.

Plant enzymes have a wider range of activity because they contain more enzymes such as the following: protease, peptidase, lipase, amylase, glucoamylase, alphagalactosidase, cellulase, hemicellulase, invertase, malt diastase, lactase, pectinase, and phytase. These enzymes are specific in their action. For example, large amounts of proteolytic enzymes can even catalyze the breakdown of the protein shell of cancer cells.

Enzyme Deficiency

Although an infant is born with the needed number of enzymes, some may be absent or at low levels and do not reach optimal levels for six to ten months. The pancreatic enzyme amylase is one of the enzymes that is at a low level at birth but is expected to be supplemented through nursing. If the baby is not nursed, raw goat milk is a very good supplement for amylase, which helps the body digest starches, but most importantly, simple sugars and carbohydrates.

Low levels of carbohydrate enzymes can lead to carbohydrate intolerance, which can progress to leaky gut syndrome. Why? Because undigested carbohydrates can feed yeast and fungi throughout the digestive system and perpetuate yeast overgrowth in the gut wall, which can contribute to perforations, letting the bacteria pass through the tight junctions and enter the blood channels that lead throughout the body. So at a very young age, you start setting the stage to develop allergies.

Most of the people I have found who have gluten intolerance or celiac disease have been people who were not nursed as babies but were bottle-fed formula and never received any amylase supplementation.

You come into the world with a storage reserve of all enzymes, except amylase. But if you are not eating foods that are supplementing your own enzymes, you will eventually deplete your "enzyme reserve." Then by the time you are 40 or 50 years old, you will discover that you are not able to break down proteins and heavy protein fibers such as in red meats. Then you start having gas and bloating and complications from that.

WHY ARE ENZYMES CRITICAL?

Enzymes are extremely important. You cannot live without them. But they require proper building blocks to be optimally effective. You have to make sure that you are getting plenty of essential minerals with your food or that you are taking enzyme supplementation. The same with amino acids. It is so critical to make sure that you have all the materials necessary. It would be like a carpenter going to build a house but forgetting the cement or nails to create the framework for the walls. This is the same thing in building your body. If you do not have all the crucial materials of enzymes, amino acids, vitamins, minerals, and oxygen, you will not maintain a healthy body with a foundation that will take you through life without disease.

Raw foods are a substantial way of replenishing the natural enzymes your body needs to keep up that reserve account for when you are eating enzyme-devoid foods at a restaurant. You want to be able to have that enzyme account in your body, so your body can call on the reserve in its bank account and continue to service the necessary digestive functions.

If you do not have the reserve when your body puts in the order for more protease, more lipase, or more maltase to digest the meal that you had in the restaurant and your bank account is empty, the body still has to force the food through the system. So it puts more trauma onto the villi and creates actual spasms within the intestinal tract while they are trying to break down and move the food because it has not been digested or broken down. This will cause inflammation that will result in bloating, upper and lower gas, restless sleep, restless legs at night, and waking up in the morning feeling fatigued because of the gases that penetrated the wall of the GI tract, entered the bloodstream, and traveled to the brain.

So how is it that we have celiac disease and gluten intolerance? It is because of the way we were raised, the way we eat or don't eat, and how we have taken care of the most critical part of our digestive system—our enzyme reserves. Are we eating foods that will replenish them? Are we supplementing with enzymes that are alive, or are we buying cheap enzymes that will not activate in the body nor have an ability to facilitate the function for which they were designed?

Enzymes are important to help clear undigested proteins out of the body, particularly the meat fibers. Undigested starches, sugars, and carbohydrates will ferment fats, turning them rancid. These toxins create a host for disease such as candida, leaky gut syndrome, brain fog, fatigue, hypoglycemia, depression, allergies, fibromyalgia, and gluten intolerance. All of these conditions can lead to more catastrophic results such as heart disease, diabetes, cancer, and progressive rheumatoid arthritis.

Enzymes Break Down Foods

Enzymes are critical to properly breaking down the foods we eat and facilitating not just the breakdown but the conversion and assimilability. They are found naturally in all forms of raw food and, as I mentioned, are present in the decaying of dead tissue.

Think about how the great chefs tenderize and add flavor to beef naturally without resorting to acids or chemicals. They use two tricks: Wet aging and dry aging. Wet aging involves wrapping a prime cut of beef with shrink wrap and allowing the natural enzymes in the beef to go to work. A family of enzymes called cathepsins may be responsible for this.

A 1990 study at the University of Nebraska found that different types of cathepsin enzymes can dramatically affect protein structures of muscles and digest proteins. Dry aging involves hanging meat out to dry for between 5 and 15 days. This is commonly practiced in many less-developed parts of the world. As the meat loses moisture with time, its weight is similarly reduced, even as its flavor becomes far superior. The only caveat is that it must be trimmed of its dried, tough exterior.[3]

The ancient Eskimos had longevity that took them well into their 70s and 80s before processed food came to their villages. Today, the northern Eskimo who lives primarily on processed food has a longevity record of between 50 and 60. Why? The ancient Eskimos lived primarily on meat and blubber. The heavy proteins and fat from the whales, seals, and caribou gave them a great deal of body heat for dealing with the cold in the wintertime. But the ancient Eskimos unknowingly also benefited from the power of the enzyme cathepsin.

They probably didn't know why, but they knew the results of hanging an animal they killed in the summertime for 10 days, sometimes longer, to allow the natural enzymes (cathepsins) to start the decomposition process within the carcass. During the winter, some tribes had caves where they would go to "cure" the meat. Such dry aging was an efficient way of predigesting and tenderizing the meat as it improved the flavor.

Another way of aging beef was to use the frozen ground as a freezer. The meat would be buried under the snow or sometimes in snow caves to allow the natural cathepsins to begin the process of digestion.

When I was a young boy, my dad was a hunter and big game guide. When we would make a kill, the animal would be hung, either in the mountains in the trees where it was taken or brought home to the farm and hung in the barn. That animal would hang for a good seven days before any processing took place. It allowed for the meat to cure, meaning it would allow all the blood to drain out of it, which would trigger cathepsin enzyme activity, which would then start the decomposition process. This practice still exists throughout the world, although it is now less prevalent.

Today, if you were to go to a feedlot where chickens, beef, pork, and other animals are raised for human consumption, you would see a very fast process in this part of meat production. The animals are run into a room where they are killed by electrical shock and are butchered immediately; the meat is then sent off to a packaging house to be packaged and sent to the stores. The meat is not hung in order to cure, so the cathepsin enzyme is unable to start the breakdown process of the fibrous tissue, making it much more difficult for the human body to digest it, particularly when our digestive systems are already compromised.

So what happens when we eat meat at night for dinner? It sits in our stomach all night long as our system works overtime to digest it. Instead of conserving its energy in self-renewal and revitalization, the body is forced to expend its precious resources in digesting very-hard-to-digest protein. Instead of making enzymes to detoxify and cleanse the body from its daily production of waste, the body must create a variety of enzymatic actions to digest the food.

Our body is designed to secrete hydrochloric acid and pepsin in the morning that starts generally an hour before awakening. That secretion may stimulate and stir the body, helping the individual to come awake.

Is changing our diet the answer to this problem? No, but that is a good place to start.

There are three things to consider:

- One, what happened to the intestinal flora of the gut?
- Two, what happened to the natural enzyme production in the body?
- Three, what is the blood pH of the person?

The answers to these three questions will give you good direction in addressing and overcoming gluten intolerance, celiac disease, food allergies, and food intolerances.

I am saddened by how our nutritional and medical communities seem to ignore the value of enzymes, realizing that everything in life would cease to exist if we didn't have any.

Enzymes are truly the most important element in the human body, and yet very little credence is given to the absence of enzymes in the process of metabolic breakdown, whether it is gluten intolerance, allergies, cancer, diabetes, or any immune-compromising condition.

In order to have proper digestion and absorption, we need to have a good level of intestinal flora. Any time an individual has undergone stress, trauma, been in a hospital for sickness or surgery, been on drugs of any kind, especially antibiotics, all of these things will compromise, if not destroy, the natural intestinal flora that maintains that balance and integrity of the gut wall and the stomach mucosal lining. The entire gastro-intestinal (GI) tract needs to have a well-furbished supply of flora to help activate and work with the enzymes.

The more we cook our foods, the fewer enzymes are going to be present. So if you eat at any fast-food restaurant, that food will have been processed a long time before you even ordered it and probably cooked at overly hot temperatures. There is no enzyme activity and no nutritional value left in that food; you are eating fiber only. If you went out and ate a cardboard box, you would probably be better off, and it might even digest better.

Enzymes have a multifaceted skill to help alleviate leaky gut. The plant-based enzymes, animal enzymes, and metabolic enzymes all play different roles in the human body. Enzymes are there to help break down food into very minute particles before it leaves the stomach, thus increasing the nutritional uptake and preventing large, undigested molecules from irritating the intestinal lining. They are also there to help digest toxins that are created in the form of gases from fermentation and putrefaction of various foods. Enzymes work through your intestines, acting like garbage collectors to remove toxins, bacteria, and damaged cells of the mucosal lining, which give the gut a clean environment of healthy cells with which to rebuild.

Some of the plant-based enzymes that are most valuable to us are bromelain and papain, found in pineapple and papaya. These have been shown over and over through research to reduce inflammation in the gut lining and other tissues in the body, helping the liver to reduce its overload.

Autism and Enzymes

Autistic children show high GI inflammation and dysfunction in both the upper and lower GI tracts. Decreased enzyme activities were reported in children with autism, and treatment of digestive problems with enzymes had a positive effect on autistic behavior.[4]

Autistic children also have a deficiency in a key detoxification pathway, according to Dr. Rosemary Waring of the School of Biosciences University of Birmingham in the UK. According to her research, autistic children are very low in sulphur in the form of sulfate, as much as 15 percent of the amount found in neurologically typical people.[5]

Toxic Overload

Food additives, flavorings, colorants, dyes, BH, BHT, TBHQ, and medications such as steroidal anti-inflammatory drugs all block the PST (the preservative tertiary butylhydroquinone) enzyme and pancreatic enzymes from carrying out their jobs.

People low in PST (phenol-sulfotransferase) enzymes or low in sulphate have problems handling environmental chemicals, some phenolic medications, or even their own body chemicals. These people are those with Parkinson's, Alzheimer's, autism, rheumatoid arthritis, chemical sensitivity, and intolerance to fats and gluten. Phenols are a necessary part of life.

A report from McFadden in 1996 stated that 2.5 percent of adults are nonmetabolizers of mucolytic drugs and even acetaminophen. These people have trouble handling environmental chemicals and become overly sensitive to medications. We see this with Parkinson's, Alzheimer's, and rheumatoid arthritis alike. The research suggests problems of sulfoxidation of the amino acid cysteine to sulfate. "Impaired sulfation has been found in many of these conditions, and preliminary data suggests that it may be important in multiple chemical sensitivities and diet responsive autism."[6]

Are enzymes the answer? They certainly are a possible answer and a support to the body in fighting to relieve symptoms of autism, Alzheimer's, Parkinson's, depression, rheumatoid arthritis, bipolar, and other diseases and disorders.

Heavy protein and starch will lie in your GI tract, primarily your stomach, at a temperature of 98.6 degrees, for 8, 10, 12 hours before the digestion really facilitates breaking it down. While it is in that alkaline environment at that temperature, it starts to ferment.

So when you wake up in the morning, instead of waking up fresh and revitalized, you start the day fatigued, groggy, and foggy minded because you still have dinner in your stomach from the night before. Even worse, gases have accumulated throughout the night from the putrefaction of the protein (from the undigested meat) and fermentation of the starches (candida and other fungi feeding on these). These gases then leach through the porous membranes of the GI tract and contribute to our toxic burden. This toxic burden is the No. 1 cause of energy depletion and liver stress.

Is coffee the answer? Or is it just a quick fix? Does it eliminate the root cause of the fatigue: toxic burden and liver overload? Or does coffee contribute to our problems? Coffee gives a wonderful jolt in the morning because it stimulates the adrenal glands to produce more adrenaline, which helps clear some of the brain fog so that folks can begin to function for a few hours, but this is just a temporary fix.

People say, "Oh, I'm not hungry; I'll just have a cup of coffee and a donut or a piece of toast and go to work." There's no good protein substance there to support the function of the body. Then by 11 o'clock, they are fatigued and "dragging." They sit behind their desk at work saying, "Oh, my goodness, I can hardly stay awake; I've got to go get another cup of coffee or soda pop." Not much difference.

The only difference between coffee and many types of soda pop is the temperature. I chuckle and smile at people who think that since they don't drink coffee, they are living a better standard of life; but they will drink beverages that have caffeine added to them, some of which have more caffeine than coffee, plus the sugar that is added to them. Those drinks are far more harmful than coffee.

Being fatigued and tired all the time is a frustrating way to live. There are so many things that we would like to do, but we are just too tired. "I would love to go outside and play with the kids, but I'm just too tired." How familiar is that?

When does disease start before it manifests itself outwardly? What do we do when going from being tired becomes aching joints, headaches, foggy thinking, dizziness, etc.? Being tired is perhaps an indication of something worse around the corner; and then when that "something worse" hits us, the next step is the doctor and medication or medications. Certainly, we want to avoid this path of pain, misery, and perhaps premature death.

The sooner we start looking at our body as a creation that needs good nutrients to function and not as a garbage dump, the sooner we will be on a path to vibrant health. We need to understand the body and what it needs to function in a healthy way. If we know what causes disease and what we can do to prevent it, we will be on the right path for overcoming fatigue.

You must be disciplined. If you are not, you will not adhere to dietary changes necessary to reverse the onset of any disease. It is all about desire, commitment, determination, and discipline, which lead to a healthy lifestyle and the positive outcome we all want.

ENDNOTES

1   Troesch B, Jing H, Laillou A, Fowler A. Aspergillus niger significantly increases iron and zinc bioavailability from phytate-rich foods. *Food Nutr Bull.* 2013 Jun;34(2 Suppl):S90-101.
2   Guggenbuhl P, Waché Y, Simoes Nunes C, Fru F. Effects of a 6-phytase on the apparent ileal digestibility of minerals and amino acids in ileorectal anastomosed pigs fed on a corn-soybean meal-barley diet. *Anim Sci.* 2012 Dec;90 Suppl 4:182-4.
3   Johnson MH, Calkins CR, Huffman RD, Johnson DD, Hargrove DD. Differences in cathepsin B + L and calcium-dependent protease activities among breed type and their relationship to beef tenderness. *J Anim Sci.* 1990 Aug;68(8):2371-9.
4   Horvath K, Perman JA. Autism and gastrointestinal symptoms. *Curr Gastroenterol Rep.* 2002 Jun;4(3):251-8.
5   Waring RH, Alberti A, et al. Sulfation deficit in "low-functioning" autistic children: a pilot study. *Biol Psychiatry.* 1999 Aug 1;46(3):420-4.
6   McFadden SA. Phenotypic variation in xenobiotic metabolism and adverse environmental response: focus on sulfur-dependent detoxification pathways. *Toxicology.* 1996 Jul 17;111(1-3):43-65.

CHAPTER 6

Diseases and Disorders
Triggered by Hybrid Gluten

H ippocrates said 2,500 years ago, "All diseases begin in the gut." Once we compromise our gut, we compromise our health and our life.

Many of our gut problems today stem from our eating foods that are not only filled with toxins but have also been hybridized or genetically modified (GMO). What is the difference?

While **hybrids are created by 'naturally'** [or specific, controlled] **crossbreeding** similar species to achieve desired traits, GM technology involves selecting genes from any living thing (similar or not) to **force the creation of DNA** that would never be found in nature. . . . **But no one knows if these foods are safe.** The only way to tell is to observe the health of those persons who consume GM foods over the long-term. Care to be a guinea pig? Neither do we! So, how do you avoid GMO foods? For now, **buy organic or foods labeled 'non-GMO.'**[1] [Emphasis in original]

GMOs, genetically modified foods, are everywhere today. The problem is that they are filled with unnatural and never-before-seen protein combinations and structures that may be a major cause of inflammation, liver stress, fatigue, and allergies.

In May of 2013, despite the fact that no genetically modified wheat has been approved for U.S. farming, a field in Oregon was found to contain Monsanto's patented Roundup Ready wheat. A report stated:

Consumers' unease with genetically modified crops, particularly those in Europe and Asia, led St. Louis-based Monsanto to end the testing of modified wheat in 2005. Many countries will not accept imports of genetically modified foods, and the United States exports half of its wheat crop. Since the announcement of the discovery of the genetically modified wheat in Oregon, Japan—one of the largest export markets for U.S. wheat growers—suspended some imports. South Korea said it would increase its inspections of U.S. wheat imports.[2]

The news report also reported that "Ninety percent of soft wheat grown in Oregon, Washington and Idaho is exported, making the states reliant on relationships with foreign markets, specifically those in Asia."[3]

In January 2014, it was reported that Monsanto's GMO wheat has advanced from "proof of concept" to "early development" stage. Monsanto's Chief Technology Officer, Robb Fraley, said, "We are still several years away from a product launch, but it is nice to see those products in the pipeline."[4] As if the hybridized wheat were not bad enough, we may have GMO wheat in just a few years!

Today's highly hybridized wheat is filled with allergenic and pro-inflammatory proteins, including proteins called gluten and gliadin.

I believe that the gluten in today's hybridized wheat is very different from the gluten in the ancient wheat (wild grasses) such as einkorn.

This chapter includes a brief overview of some of the health- and life-compromising diseases and disorders that are related to problems in the gut.

ALLERGIES

Almost every person over the age of 30 has some allergy or sensitivity to some types of foods, even foods that are healthy.

People have had allergy tests and have been told that they were allergic to eggs; but when tested further, they discovered that they were actually allergic to the fat in the egg yolk but not to the protein in the egg white.

Other people have allergies to yeast, which is rich in B vitamins. If you are deficient in B vitamins, then you run the risk of developing Type 1 or Type 2 diabetes, and certainly you will have hypoglycemia at an exaggerated level.

Allergies can create considerable inflammation in the body, which then unleashes a host of other problems. For example, asthma has been referred to as an allergy, and arthritis can also be classified as an allergy because it is related to inflammation, which is the root cause of many chronic diseases.

A 2004 WebMD Health News article begins, "Allergies and asthma may start in your gut. Upset the gut's natural mix of helpful bacteria and fungi, and allergies and asthma may develop."[5]

ASPERGER'S SYNDROME

Asperger's syndrome is often considered to be a mild form of autism. It affects nonverbal communication and behavioral development in children, and its main symptom is that children have significant trouble in social situations, although there is a wide variety of symptoms.

We seem to have a difficult time dealing with children who are "differently-abled." Take the case of Temple Grandin. Her parents were told she was autistic and should be institutionalized. She didn't speak until she was nearly four years old. But Temple figured out that she thought differently, in images, and fought her way to a bachelor's degree in psychology, and master's and doctoral degrees in animal science. She is probably the world's most famous (and successful) person with Asperger's, which she is now considered to be. She designed the facilities in which half the cattle in the U.S. are handled and has been a professor at Colorado State University for two decades.

On her website, Grandin is quoted as saying, "One of the problems today is for a kid to get any special services in school, they have to have a label. The problem with autism is you've got a spectrum that goes from Einstein down to someone with no language."[6]

AUTISM

Autism is a disorder that is marked by impaired cognitive development and functioning in children, leading to problems with social interaction, communication skills, and behavior patterns. Autism was thought to be genetic, but the most recent studies are showing that there may be environmental factors and definitely food factors that are influencing this condition.

According to the organization Autism Speaks, the largest study of its kind was conducted at Sweden's Karolinska Institute on autism and celiac disease. While the researchers found no link between autism and celiac disease, they did find a strong association between autism and the presence of antibodies to gluten. Gastroenterologist Alessio Fasano commented, "In the past, we have had the believers and the nonbelievers when it came to the role of gluten in autism. Hopefully, this paper can clarify, once and for all, that a subset of those with autism has gluten sensitivity, a condition triggered by gluten but distinct from celiac disease."[7]

The alarming rate of growth of autism in the United States and worldwide and the increased awareness of parents and many medical practitioners is starting to provoke more and more research and debate. Various studies, particularly those conducted by alternative practitioners, suggest that there may be a link between autism and food allergies, specifically gluten, a protein found in barley, wheat, and rye. These allergies may be responsible for making autism become worse.

Many of the mental symptoms such as brain fog are often mistakenly associated with children's psychiatric disorders. However, gluten intolerance and celiac disease create brain fog, so perhaps the symptoms are caused by a combination of a reaction to gluten and their autistic behaviors, which are intensified because of the gluten.

Children display more mental symptoms to gluten intolerance because their brains are still developing, making them more susceptible. Adults show more physical symptoms because their brains are not in a developmental stage.

Parents often recognize a behavior change in their children when they stop eating gluten, but does this mean that gluten intolerance causes autism? Not likely. It is more likely that gluten intolerance exacerbates the autistic symptoms and behavior.

How many generations could it take to modify the metabolic process in the human body? How long can you saturate the body with hidden chemicals and genetically modified food molecules with chemicals to withstand pesticides and herbicides without changing behavior? How many of our genetically engineered foods have excess chromosomes that the human body tries to digest but cannot identify? How many people have adequate secretion of hydrochloric acid, pepsin, and the other enzymes necessary for proper digestion and assimilation? How can the liver overloaded with toxins promote the metabolic processes of cleansing the blood and tissue pathways of inorganic material and toxic pathogens?

CANDIDA

What is Candida? The most common fungus species in humans is *Candida albicans,* a form of yeast. A small amount normally lives in the intestines and other parts of the body and aids in digestion and nutrient absorption. A problem occurs when there is an overgrowth of candida, which compromise the walls of the intestines, contributing to leaky gut syndrome, and penetrate the bloodstream, releasing toxins into the body.

Many factors can lead to a yeast overgrowth in the human body. Antibiotics, which are used to kill harmful bacteria, also kill the beneficial bacteria in an individual's intestines. Once the friendly flora in the gut is drastically impaired, this sets the stage for opportunistic yeast overgrowth. In addition, a weakened immune system leaves the body more susceptible to an overgrowth of candida.

Gluten intolerance more than likely encourages the overgrowth of candida. If left untreated, gluten intolerance and/or celiac disease will wreak havoc with the immune system. I have never met a person who had rheumatoid arthritis who when we tested did not have either a high level of gluten intolerance or one of the stages of celiac disease and didn't even realize it. They were still eating wheat bread in different forms and wondering why they now would eat wheat bread but feel weak, wiped out, and bloated for two or three days afterwards.

Gluten intolerance impairs the secretion of enzymes, reducing the effects of digestion and absorption and creating more fermentation. Gluten intolerance and candida go hand in hand.

When the larger, undigested food molecules and/or undigested food bacteria become rancid in the gut from fermentation, lack of enzymes, and lack of proper acid balance, the body begins developing an overgrowth of the natural native yeasts and fungi. The overgrowth causes fermentation in the gut, creating more fungal waste products and toxins; other forms of food waste that are undigested will also contribute to more toxic fermentation.

Many folks would not care to think about a fungal life cycle. It consumes or "ferments" starches and sugars and then it defecates, just as any other living organism. The problem: there are no toilets in your gut, and so these potentially toxic fungal waste products leach into your intestines and into your blood, and there is little you can do to prevent this. Eliminating GMO foods and gluten from your diet will slow fungal growth. Pomegranates are an example of a natural food with anti-fungal properties. A 2012 study at the State University of Moringa in Brazil found that pomegranate might be "useful for treating candidiasis."[8]

Another study at the Aligappa University in 2013 concluded that, ". . . pomegranate was shown to inhibit the formation of biofilms by *Staphylococcus aureus, methicillin resistant S. aureus, Escherichia coli,* and *Candida albicans.*"[9]

Practices related to gluten intolerance are primarily structured around diet restrictions. For example, eliminating sugars, starches, hybrid grains, and other GMO or processed foods reduces the inflammation and retards **candida overgrowth**. While this may be a good start, it is not a permanent solution.

In the 1950s and '60s, people started to become aware of the word "candida," and it became one of the most talked-about health problems. However, the medical profession called candida a phony disease that quack practitioners, naturopaths, chiropractors, and homeopaths had invented. Now they have claimed it as theirs to the degree that they have made drugs to treat it.

This yeast fungus can be linked to many different health problems besides candida, like allergies, depression, poor memory, digestive problems, leaky gut syndrome, hypoglycemia, fibromyalgia, and Epstein Barr virus.

In an article written for the *Natural Health News and Community*, Dr. Jeffrey McCombs writes:

> Hwp-1, also known as Hyphal Wall Protein-1, is an amino acid within the cell wall of *Candida albicans* that enables Candida cells to attach to the intestinal cells. The sequence of amino acids that make up Hwp-1 are identical or highly similar to the proteins, α-gliadin and γ-gliadin found in gluten (wheat, barley, rye) products. When Candida attaches to the intestinal wall, the body's immune system responds.

> The cells of the immune system don't recognize the Hwp-1 as being separate from the intestinal cell. It sees them as both being a part of the same foreign material. From that point on, it can then target both substances either together or separately.

> Due to the similarities between Hwp-1 and gluten proteins, this can lead to autoimmune diseases like Celiac Disease where the immune system attacks the cells of the intestine when gluten products are ingested. This autoimmune process has been implicated in a host of other inflammatory conditions and patterns throughout the body. Over 150 medical conditions have been reported to have an increased prevalence among gluten sensitive individuals. Long-term inflammation of the intestinal tract can also lead to malabsorption syndromes, anemia, immunosuppression, nervous system disorders, infertility, inflammatory bowel disorders, and cancers.[10]

In the 1950s and '60s, the hybridization of wheat and the use of chemicals on our food crops were widespread. The chemical companies were well under way creating herbicides to kill weeds and grasses to give the farmers better yields and were looking at how they could hybridize and genetically modify different crops, since they had become so successful in hybridizing wheat.

All those pesticides, herbicides, and preservatives that are put on salad greens in stores to keep them from wilting go into the gut and mix with any sugar present, thus promoting the overgrowth of the candida and more toxic gases that compromise the health of the body.

Then instead of waking up fresh in the morning, you wake up fatigued and groggy and can't remember where you left your car keys. Gases that have passed through the porous membranes of the GI tract from the candida overgrowth cause more fermentation from the meat, starches, and proteins that have been in the gut for 8 to 10 hours during the night, then leach into the bloodstream, reducing the oxygen in the blood that flows to the brain, causing more fatigue in the morning.

The answer is to change your diet! It is also highly important to take pre- and probiotics to build the intestinal flora. This is crucial for any health condition, irrespective of whether it is gluten intolerance, celiac disease, or candida, which generally gains its foothold from the lack of intestinal flora not being properly supported from pre- and probiotics.

CELIAC DISEASE

Celiac disease is a direct reaction to the gliadin, which is a gluten protein found in wheat, barley, and rye. Some argue that oats are contaminated by wheat.[11] The inflammation irritates and usually damages the inner lining of the small intestine. It is a little different from gluten intolerance in that it is a more advanced breakdown of the autoimmune system that may be caused from the onset of gluten intolerance.

Presently, there is no known cure for celiac disease or gluten intolerance other than diet management.

Some of the symptoms that indicate that there is a problem are a tender stomach and rashes in different places on the body such as across the abdomen, on the lower torso, or on thighs running down over the shins. It looks like psoriasis but may actually be caused by celiac disease.

How can we identify the conditions? Celiac disease can affect genetically predisposed people of any age. Some of the symptoms that are often ignored are fatigue, diarrhea, weight loss, and/or weight gain. Many times the weight gain is from bloating, not so much from getting fatter, but from bloating and retaining fluid.

There are various levels of celiac disease, 1, 2, 3, and 4, with 4 being the most severe.

In Level 1 people have fatigue, anemia, occasional abdominal discomfort with a little bloating, distention, and excessive gas that will vary from day to day based on what they are eating.

Celiac disease is considered a permanent disorder, and its effects can change from time to time based on eating habits and volume and choices of foods.

In Level 2 Celiac disease can raise havoc on other organs in the body, causing liver problems and constipation because the bowel has become dysfunctional and is unable to break down and absorb the nutrients. Both Levels 1 and 2 have a lot of fluid retention, which causes fat accumulation.

Many other symptoms that develop are bone and joint pain, diarrhea, easy bruising, flatulence, fluid retention, foul-smelling stools, gastritis, gastrointestinal discomfort, overall weakness, fatigue, increased amount of fat in the stools, infertility, persistent hunger, mouth sores, irritability, malnutrition, and often deficiencies of vitamins B12, D, and K. Depression is also very common.

Levels 3 and 4 deal with weight loss, which encompasses muscle wasting, cramping, muscle weakness, nausea, vomiting, nose bleeding, stomach discomfort, pale in appearance, slight lactose intolerance, osteoporosis, panic attacks, and/or red urine. Skin rashes are very common from Levels 2 to 4; and the more severe the Celiac disease becomes, the more severe the rashes become.

With advanced Celiac disease, neuropathy symptoms start appearing with weaknesses in different parts of the body, particularly the legs. Aching in the hip joints, pelvis area, knees, and shoulders is very typical. These conditions are often diagnosed as fibromyalgia, Crohn's disease, irritable bowel syndrome, or even candida.

Many of these symptoms manifest in different levels of Celiac disease that can mimic or mask other diseases. Some people think they are dealing with Celiac disease, when in reality, cancer was the underlying cause and Celiac disease was a byproduct.

What about children? After hundreds of years of eating wheat, children are now developing gluten intolerance, celiac disease, irritable bowel syndrome, colitis, food sensitivities, and allergies.

Celiac disease retards growth, which sometimes is labeled as juvenile onset dwarfism; but it has nothing to do with the pituitary gland. As children start growing into puberty, the symptoms of Celiac disease sometimes just go away, perhaps as their digestive system strengthens. Maybe they started eating better food, better enzymes, or started taking vitamins such as B3, B6, and B12, which are essential for children to combat the disease.

When left untreated, Celiac disease can increase to the point of developing heart disease and cancer. Celiac disease is directly connected to intestinal lymphoma and other forms of cancer, especially adrenal carcinoma of the small intestines, pharynx, and esophagus, as well as ulcers in the small intestine.

Keratosis pilaris, also referred to as "chicken skin," is where little bumps form on the back of the arms. When you run your hand over the skin, it feels bumpy. This indicates a vitamin A and fatty acid deficiency and the inability to metabolize fat, which often damages the gut.

Other symptoms are brain fog and persistent fatigue, which often follow a meal that contains gluten. Other symptoms include neurological problems such as dizziness or a feeling of being off balance.

Hormones can be greatly disturbed with celiac disease or gluten intolerance, which decreases the production of estrogen in women and contributes to PMS and infertility.

Gluten and highly hybridized grains can also trigger the onset of autoimmune diseases such as Hashimoto's disease that affects the thyroid. Low thyroid activity can further add to our fatigue Other immune disorders created by the unnatural proteins in today's highly hybridized wheat include rheumatoid arthritis, ulcerative colitis, lupus, psoriasis, scleroderma, or multiple sclerosis and are all associated with advanced stages of gluten intolerance and celiac disease.

Those suffering migraine headaches should first check for food allergies and sensitivities, as well as for gluten intolerance.

Anyone diagnosed with chronic fatigue syndrome or fibromyalgia should start asking questions, because more than likely the problem will be gluten intolerance.

Watch for inflammation and swelling in the joints, fingers, knees, and hips; and watch for mood issues such as anxiety, depression, mood swings, and attention deficit/hyperactivity disorder (ADHD). Wheat gliadin ultimately attacks the villi lining the small intestine, causing diarrhea and/or constipation, pain, anemia, and fatigue.

Are the medical tests for gluten intolerance conclusive? Not likely, because gluten intolerance, celiac disease, fibromyalgia, Crohn's disease, irritable bowel syndrome, and diverticulitis can all be interrelated and cause problems at the same time.

People can also develop Celiac disease from eating grains like rye and barley; but the modern hybridized wheat, is the main culprit with its changed chemical structure.

Gluten intolerance has dramatically increased in the United States over the past 50 years. Celiac disease affects an estimated 1 in 133 people in the U.S. alone. It is considered a hereditary disorder, because a person must have a genetic predisposition for it to develop it.

Your chances of being diagnosed with it jump from 1 in 133 to 1 in 39 if a cousin, aunt, or uncle has it and 1 in 22 if a member of your immediate family has it.

Interestingly, celiac disease is far less common in people of African, Hispanic, and Asian descent: just 1 in 236. This disease is also more likely to occur in combination with lactose intolerance, as well as Type 1 diabetes.[12]

However, a lot more is involved with celiac than just being an inherited disorder. It seems to be caused by many factors, both inherited and environmental, including the following:

- Inheritance (genes)
- Enzyme deficiency
- Leaky gut syndrome
- Poor nutrition due to eating the Standard American Diet (SAD)
- Damage to the intestinal lining
- Hybridization of wheat
- Genetically modified foods

When someone has the predisposition to develop celiac, it seems to be triggered by something in the diet that activates it.

Joseph Murray, MD, of the Mayo Clinic saw about one celiac patient per year in Iowa beginning in 1988. He noticed that by 1997, 100 patients were diagnosed yearly at the hospital where he worked. He figured that because they were looking for celiac now, they were finding it more often.

Then a rare treasure fell into his hands after joining the Mayo Clinic. Blood samples from Air Force recruits in the early 1950s had been frozen after streptococcus broke out in the barracks. The samples were donated to the University of Minnesota, and Dr. Murray's team started testing for gluten antibodies, expecting to find a small percentage.

But the results were much lower, indicating that celiac disease was very low among these young men. So the team compared results with:

. . . two recently collected sets from Olmestead County, Minn. One blood sample set matched the birth years of the airmen. Elderly men were four times likelier to have celiac disease than their contemporaries tested 50 years earlier. The second set matched the ages of the airmen at the time their blood was drawn. Today's young men are 4.5 times likelier to have celiac disease than the 1950s recruits.

This tells us that whatever has happened with celiac disease has happened since 1950, but the increase has affected both the young and old suggesting that something happened in a pervasive fashion from the environmental perspective.[13]

A Mayo Clinic article suggests several possibilities for this four-fold increase in celiac disease since 1950. Perhaps the "hygiene hypothesis" where our environment is so clean the immune system is underutilized and attacks the body. "Another possible culprit is the 21st century diet. Although overall wheat consumption hasn't increased, the ways wheat is processed and eaten have changed dramatically. . . . Modern wheat also differs from older strains because of hybridization."[14]

The Mayo Clinic did a study in 2009 to see if undiagnosed CD [celiac disease] had changed in the last 50 years. The study reports: "The prevalence of undiagnosed CD seems to have increased dramatically in the United States during the past 50 years."[15]

Similar results were found in a study from Finland in 2007, where the conclusion was, "The total prevalence of coeliac disease seems to have doubled in Finland during the past two decades, and the increase cannot be attributed to the better detection rate. The environmental factors responsible for the increasing prevalence of the disorder are issues for further studies."[16]

Most people believe they are eating healthy if they are eating "whole-grain" wheat and don't know that one slice of whole wheat bread raises the blood sugar more than a candy bar or a can of soda. Dr. Davis showed that the glycemic index of whole wheat bread is 72, while the glycemic index of a Mars bar is 68![17]

What do we eat for breakfast? Maybe we eat bacon and eggs but with toast, waffles, pancakes, bagels, or muffins. Lunch may often be a sandwich or a hamburger on a bun. Dinner may include bread or biscuits and some cake or pastry as dessert. We are smothered in hybridized, dwarf wheat, and it is killing us.

I like this statement by Dr. Mark Hyman: "The end of your fork is more powerful than the bottom of your pill bottle."[18] Are we digging our graves with a fork?

DEMENTIA AND ALZHEIMER'S

Are gluten intolerance and wheat-related autoimmune reactions linked with accelerated cognitive decline with age?

Let's examine the data:

It is very sobering to think that 20 years ago, dementia was considered to be just an old people's disease. Today, the elderly population, those age 65 years and older, is expected to double by 2030. With this rapid growth in the number of older people, prevention and treatment of dementia and Alzheimer's will take on growing importance.

One of the biggest concerns we have worldwide is dementia, particularly because the decline in memory and other cognitive functions that characterize this condition also leads to a loss of independence that has a wide range of impacts on individuals' and families' health care systems and other insurance programs for elderly adults.

Worldwide, more than 36 million people have been formally diagnosed with dementia today, and 115 million are predicted by 2050. It has been determined that only 1 out of 5 people have gone for formal diagnosis, and some health care providers say that it is closer to 1 out of 50.

In high-income countries, only 20 to 50 percent of the people with dementia are receiving primary care. The total estimated costs of dementia in the U.S. alone in 2010 was $604 billion. If dementia were a country, it would be the world's 18th largest economy.

We see that people 71 and older have a 13.9 percent rate, comprising about 3.4 million individuals in the U.S. in 2002. The corresponding values for Alzheimer's disease were 9.7 percent rate and 2.4 million individuals. Dementia prevalence increased with age from 5 percent of those age 71 to 79 years, to 37.4 percent for those age 90 and older.[19]

We look at some of the statistics in other countries like Australia, and they are staggering. In 2010 there were over 321,600 Australians living with dementia. This number is expected to increase by one third to 400,000 in less than 10 years.

Without a medical breakthrough, the number of people with dementia is expected to be almost 900,000 in Australia by 2050. If every person who showed symptoms of dementia today were to go in and have a formal diagnosis, that number of 900,000 predicted for 2050 would appear in 2015. Each week there are 1,700 new cases of dementia in Australia, approximately 1 person every 6 minutes. This is expected to grow by 7,400 new cases each week by 2050.

The prevalence of dementia is reaching down into the younger generations. Nearly 25,000 people in Australia are diagnosed with younger-onset dementia, a diagnosis of dementia under the age of 65. This is including people as young as 30. Three in ten people over the age of 85 and almost one in ten people over 65 have dementia in Australia, and an estimated 1.2 million Australians are caring for someone with dementia.[20]

In a 2012 Natural Health Advisory article, Elaine Fawcett, N.T.P., writes:
Think that morning bagel or pasta dinner is no big deal? Think again. Studies show eating gluten can cause brain disorders that could ultimately raise your risk of memory loss, dementia symptoms, and Alzheimer's. . . . a gluten-free diet is an important consideration when it comes to brain health.

Most Gluten-Intolerant People Have No Digestive Complaints
Many people think gluten intolerance or celiac disease means suffering from digestive complaints. The truth is only a minority of people with gluten intolerance or celiac disease complain of digestive issues or pain, and some have no symptoms whatsoever. Nevertheless, for those with undiagnosed gluten intolerance, gluten can silently wreak havoc in the brain [and gut] for years or decades before symptoms, including loss of memory and cognition, begin to manifest.

Some Research Shows Link Between Gluten and Dementia Symptoms
Although studies showing a direct connection between gluten intolerance and dementia are scant, some insight exists. . . .

Although little research has been done directly linking gluten intolerance with dementia symptoms and Alzheimer's, gluten's effects on neurology in general are more established. Gluten can profoundly affect the brain and nervous system and has been shown to present as an exclusively neurological disease in many people.

Gluten's Effects on Brain May Raise Risk of Dementia Symptoms
In one study, researchers linked gluten to neurological problems,

including ADHD, in 51 percent of children with gluten sensitivity. Other studies show gluten can trigger both inflammation and autoimmune attacks in the brain, both of which damage and destroy brain tissue and cause such symptoms as brain fog, autism spectrum disorders, learning disabilities, and loss of memory and cognition. . . .

Due to highly developed communication between the brain and the digestive system, the brain's own inflammatory system responds to inflammation in the gut. . . . and hence raise the risk of dementia symptoms.

Gluten-free Diet Improves Outcome of Dementia Symptoms for Some

If symptoms of memory loss or dementia become an issue, a gluten-free diet and other dietary strategies can't hurt, and it's potential for helping is statistically relevant. However, it is even better to prevent memory loss and reduce the risk of Alzheimer's by finding out if there is an immune response to gluten. Tests commonly performed in doctor's offices have a low accuracy rate. The best test is to remove gluten from your diet for at least a month and see how you feel (although some people take as long as nine months to notice benefit because gluten's effects on the immune system are long-lasting).[21]

To help reverse the incidence of dementia, we need to change our diets and eliminate products made with modern hybrid wheat and any other hybrid or genetically modified grains.

DIABETES

Another common issue tied to gluten intolerance is diabetes, which is a lifelong high level of sugar in the blood. It can be caused by too little insulin, resistance to insulin, or both. Gluten intolerance causes a pancreas dysfunction, which is the inability to regulate insulin and glucose.

Gluten sensitivity disorders and diabetes are both autoimmune diseases and have similar symptoms, and both can cause inflammation that may result in significant damage to the body.

People with diabetes should check their sensitivity to gluten, and people with celiac disease and other gluten sensitivity disorders should check their blood sugar levels.

FIBROMYALGIA

In a 2013 article, Suzanne Elvidge reported:

According to the American Chronic Pain Society, fibromyalgia syndrome is one of the most common chronic pain conditions in the world. The main symptoms of fibromyalgia syndrome are pain and tenderness across the body, with severe tiredness and problems with sleep—around 90% . . . will have problems with sleep. Because the symptoms of fibromyalgia syndrome are very varied and . . . can be quite difficult to diagnose, the statistics for people with the disorder can vary quite widely, and the figures can often be based on estimates rather than actual numbers.

How Many People Worldwide Have Fibromyalgia Syndrome?

According to the National Fibromyalgia Association, 3-6% of the world's population has fibromyalgia syndrome. With a projected world population of 6,816,322,780 in April 2010 . . . , this estimate would mean that somewhere around 200 million to 400 million people worldwide have fibromyalgia syndrome.[22]

More than 12 million Americans have fibromyalgia. Most of them are women ranging in age from 25 to 60. Women are 10 times more likely to get this disease than men.[23]

Fibromyalgia patients often complain of heart stress and anxiety, arrhythmia, palpitations, heart pain, and inflammation. It can occur after a series of minor injuries, overuse, or abuse of muscles and nerves, making them weak and causing pain.

Fibromyalgia is also considered the overuse syndrome with a lot of anxiety. Every emotional upset impacts the level of pain. Hypoxia, which is low oxygen levels, is present in the painful muscles. Unoxygenated blood is caused by stress, poor diet, and lack of exercise and causes pain, disease, and premature death.

One of the most prominent features of fibromyalgia is fatigue, which is also a symptom of chronic fatigue syndrome, hypothyroidism, food allergies, gluten intolerance, celiac disease, POTS (postural orthostatic tachycardia syndrome), depression, and manic depressant conditions.

Today we are eating out of fast-food restaurants and boxes of prepared foods to make life easy and more convenient, which means we are eating foods devoid of enzymes and minerals. Processed foods are enzyme dead, and without enzymes, minerals cannot be used by the body. You can't make hormones, build immunity, or have good digestion without the proper enzymes.

Food allergies and intolerances, especially wheat gluten sensitivity, seem to be factors in fibromyalgia. Try going wheat-free for a month and see if it helps.

Many diseases have many common symptoms that cause misdiagnosis. Inflammation in the muscles creates fibromyalgia symptoms, celiac symptoms, POTS symptoms, arthritic hypothyroidism, and rheumatism.

GLYCATION/AGES

By increasing blood sugar more than cubes of white sugar, modern hybridized wheat causes accelerated aging of your tissues without your even realizing it.

When sugar and protein molecules combine, they form a tangled, tough, and inflexible connective tissue called "glycation." This tissue leads to the wrinkling of the skin; and where flexibility is vital, this inelastic, tough connective tissue is very damaging to internal organs. These glycated tissues produce Aged Glycation End-products (AGEs), which produce large numbers of damaging free radicals.

These protein molecules collectively disrupt your body from the organs to the bloodstream and arteries. AGEs accumulate and form clumps of debris that the body cannot digest or eliminate.

The formation of AGEs is an irreversible process, causing structural and functional changes in protein, leading to various complications in diabetes, angiopathy, neuropathy, light neuropathy, and retinopathy. It also leads to various complications of diabetes.

Consuming bread from processed hybrid wheat will trigger dramatic blood sugar spikes. For example, consuming one slice of white bread will raise blood sugar almost twice as much as chomping down 4 sugar cubes! And all that blood sugar is not healthy. Think about why diabetics go blind or have limbs amputated because of chronically high blood sugar.

The high blood sugar spikes caused by wheat can also contribute to the formation of cataracts, dementia, hardened arteries, and other degenerative diseases of aging. Sugar is very reactive and binds with proteins to render them deformed and permanently damaged (AGEs). The older you get, the more deformed sugar-protein complexes (AGEs) can be found in your kidneys, eyes, liver, skin, and other glands. The issue is whether two or more decades of eating the wrong food has aged you faster than you might be genetically programmed to age had you eaten better foods.

Beware of the age-accelerating effects of high blood glucose. Foods that don't result in quick sugar spikes from low glycemic foods are breads and crackers made from flax seed or einkorn, coconut flour, lentil flours, and non-grain flours that are known to not cause a rapid rise in blood sugar levels.

But watch out for those wheat bagels, muffins, and breads, because hybrid wheat can make a blood glucose level rise, at least in some people, and could make you age faster. It would be interesting to speculate which product would win in a contest between modern hybrid wheat and ice cream in raising your blood sugar.

Inflammation is not caused by one condition. It is not about just having an allergy to gluten. It's the whole process that takes place in forming inflammation. Raising the blood glucose is just one problem that creates allergy or autoimmune disorders because of the compounding of the advanced glycation process.

People say, "I was fine until a year ago. Now, all of a sudden, I start to eat something, feel bloated, and can't eat as much. I feel foggy and my head is not clear; I can't respond and I can't remember." Why is this happening? It is called, "filling the bucket" of your body with one spoonful or one forkful of bad food at a time, drinking bad water or other liquids one drink at a time, and breathing air that is toxic, one breath at a time. It is all cumulative, and when the bucket is filled up, it starts spilling over with a host of other problems.

The body is now saturated, and if the pancreas is the weakest part of the body, diabetes manifests. If the weakest part of the body happens to be the joints, then arthritis manifests. If the weakest part of the body is the colon, then irritable bowel syndrome, Crohn's, or celiac disease will manifest.

INFLAMMATION

Our body's reaction to genetically modified gluten and wheat proteins cause the single largest factor for disease: Chronic excess inflammation. According to William Meggs of East Carolina University, "Inflammation may well turn out to be the elusive holy grail of medicine, the single phenomenon that holds the key to sickness and health."

Inflammation comes from the Latin word *inflammo,* meaning, "Set alight, I ignite." Just like fire can be both good and bad, inflammation can be both healthy and unhealthy.

Healthy Inflammation

Moderate inflammation is a healthy immune system response and one of the body's tools for healing and fighting infection. It is how the body protects itself. Immune cells rush to the site of damage or infection, bringing redness, swelling, heat, and pain. Inflammation is like a wall or a protective shield that helps to stop further movement that might cause more damage. This in turn also enables the body to begin the healing process by removing harmful bacteria, including damaged cells, irritants, and pathogens and opens the pathways, allowing for healing nutrients to begin the repair.

In cases like a sprained ankle, the body releases antibodies to start the swelling process, primarily to immobilize the damaged ankle and highlight the pain, so you won't put all your weight back on the ankle and increase the damage. It's a warning indicator that there is something wrong and that you need to pay attention to the damaged area. We have probably never fully realized the value of inflammation and the important role it plays in the body.

Unhealthy Inflammation

The war that rages within us is the dark side of inflammation. If the body becomes "stuck" in an inflammatory mode, it is called chronic inflammation and may be linked to diseases such as coronary heart disease, diabetes, fibromyalgia, cystic fibrosis, Crohn's Disease, irritable bowel syndrome, and cancer. Inflammation is a double-edged sword and can be the cause of pain, disease, and premature aging or be the body's biggest protection mechanism.

An autoimmune disorder like arthritis is a sign of an immune system that is attacking its host—your body—instead of harmful invaders like bacteria. It is "friendly fire" because your own immune cells are attacking the healthy tissue (such as the cartilage in your joints in the case of arthritis). The immune system becomes confused and sees normal tissue as harmful pathogens or irritants. It then automatically triggers an inflammatory response to capture those irritants and pathogens that are believed to be harmful and eliminate them from the body. The destruction of healthy tissue—known as autoimmune disorders—begins by the body being provoked by inflammation.

What has caused the increase in celiac disease, chronic inflammation, and auto-immune disorders? Why were they not heard of 100 years ago, 50 years ago, or even 25 years ago? Why the dramatic increase in just the last couple of decades?

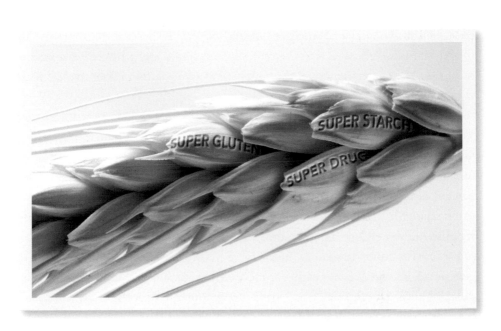

Inflammatory Role of Highly Hybridized Wheat

As mentioned in an earlier chapter, this quote from Dr. Mark Hyman, MD, deserves repeating. He warns about modern wheat and the breads that are made from "dwarf wheat plants with much higher amounts of starch and gluten and many more chromosomes coding for all sorts of new odd proteins."[24] Dr. Hyman calls dwarf wheat a "Frankenfood" and says that it drives obesity, diabetes, etc., in three ways:

1. It contains the **Super Starch** amylopectin A that is super fattening.
2. It contains a form of **Super Gluten** that is super-inflammatory.
3. It contains forms of a **Super Drug** that are super addictive and makes you crave and eat more.[25]

Dr. William Davis explains that changes from all this hybridization resulted in wheat that "expresses a higher quantity of genes for gluten proteins that are associated with celiac disease."[26]

Research on Inflammation

A study at Pennington Biomedical Research Center in Baton Rouge, Louisiana, showed an association between fitness, fatness, and total white blood cell count. They found that overweight men have higher inflammatory markers than men of the same age who are not overweight. There is also an increase in the white blood cell levels that are typically and traditionally linked to coronary heart disease in overweight and obese men. This same pattern is very typical with women as well.[27]

The scientists at the Fred Hutchinson Cancer Research Center in Seattle, Washington, found that post-menopausal, overweight, or obese women who lost 5 percent or more of their body weight had measurable falls in levels of inflammation markers, as well as decreased neutrophil counts. Team leader Ann McTiernan, MD, PhD, said both obesity and inflammation have been shown to be related to several types of cancer, and this study shows that if you reduce weight, you also reduce inflammation and cancer risk as well.[28]

Scientists from Stanford University in California have identified 15 new genetic regions associated with coronary artery disease that are the result of plaque building up in heart vessel walls. According to one of the study's authors, Tim Assimes, some people may be born predisposed to the development of coronary atherosclerosis because they inherited mutations in some key genes related to inflammation.[29]

We need to protect our bodies by learning what the body needs to stay healthy and stop heart-damaging inflammation through diet and exercise.

Inflammation and Autoimmune Diseases

There are many different types of inflammation related to autoimmune diseases:

- **Rheumatoid arthritis:** Inflammation of the joints and the surrounding tissue and sometimes organs such as the heart
- **Ankylosing spondylitis:** Inflammation that causes vertebrae of the spine to fuse together, possibly causing deformity
- **Celiac disease:** Caused by gluten intolerance that damages the intestinal lining that may result in weight loss, malnutrition, and diarrhea
- **Crohn's disease:** A type of inflammatory bowel disease with abdominal pain and diarrhea
- **Fibromyalgia:** Widespread musculoskeletal pain that brings fatigue, affects memory and sleep, and causes mood changes; can manifest anywhere in the body, even if the existence of inflammation is unclear, making it difficult to diagnose, simply because the pain moves to different parts of the body; often misdiagnosed as early stages of arthritis or rheumatoid arthritis

- **Graves' disease:** The leading cause of hyperthyroidism, a condition in which the thyroid gland produces excessive hormones
- **Psoriasis:** An immune-related disorder of the skin, causing red, scaly patches and plaque
- **Lupus:** An inflammatory disease that occurs when the body's immune system attacks tissues and organs and can affect skin, kidneys, blood cells, brain, heart, and lungs
- **Vasculitis:** A disorder of inflammation, which eventually destroys blood vessels of both arteries and veins

Dangerous Anti-inflammatory Drugs

What does the medical profession offer for these inflammatory conditions? Often the first prescription is for NSAIDs: non-steroidal anti-inflammatory drugs. Prominent NSAIDS are ibuprofen, aspirin, and naproxen.

People are cautioned to not use these drugs long term without being under the supervision of a doctor because there is a risk of stomach ulcers and even severe and life-threatening hemorrhages. NSAIDs may also worsen asthma symptoms and cause kidney damage. With the exception of aspirin, these drugs can also increase the risk of stroke and myocardial infarction (heart attacks).

The pharmaceutical drug medically known as paracetamol or acetaminophen can reduce pain associated with inflammatory conditions; but it has negligible anti-inflammatory effects, so it is not considered an NSAID. It may be ideal for those wishing to treat just the pain, if they don't mind allowing the inflammation to run its course.

Traditional corticosteroids are a class of steroid hormones produced by the body in the adrenal cortex (the outer portion of the adrenal gland). Corticosteroids are synthesized in laboratories, added to medications, and used to regulate inflammation. There are two types: glucocorticoids like cortisol and mineral corticoids like aldosterone.

Synthetic glucocorticoids are prescribed for inflammation of the joints, arthritis, temporal arteries, dermatitis, inflammatory bowel disease, systemic lupus, hepatitis, asthma, allergic reactions, and sarcoidosis. Topical creams and ointments are often prescribed for inflammation of the skin, eyes, lungs, bowels, and nose.

Toxins and Inflammation

With its huge payload of "unfamiliar proteins," modern wheat contributes not only to inflammation but to our toxic burden.

Our liver is constantly working to filter, process, and detoxify all of the food and chemicals we ingest. Eventually, we reach the point that the liver is unable to keep up with the constant onslaught of toxic waste. All of the toxins that come from food, pesticides, herbicides, chemicals, fertilizers, sprays, stabilizers, and preservatives, and the fungus or yeast overgrowth that is triggered by them, accumulate in the body. Then we wonder why we have dysfunctional body systems causing headaches and chronic fatigue.

A toxic overload will manifest in some form or another to tell us there is a problem, but too many people don't recognize that the body is giving a warning and continue to eat the same things and wonder what is wrong.

Depression, ADHD, and anxiety are typical of what we don't understand; and when we run to the doctor, he says, "Oh, it's genetic; you must have inherited it."

That is like saying that because my mother had arthritis, I am going to have arthritis. My mother was starting down the path toward arthritis as a child and was beginning to suffer the effects of the disease by the time she was 26 years old, and she died from rheumatoid arthritis and many other complications. Does her plight mean that I have to have arthritis? My grandfather and my uncles died from cancer, so does that mean I have to die from cancer because it is supposedly genetic?

We all have the ability to change our destiny by taking charge of it, by being responsible for our health.

If we take a serious look at inflammation or at any type of degenerative condition, perhaps we can start to understand what causes it and how we can prevent and/or overcome it. Perhaps we need to look at how modern "miracle" wheat is contributing to it.

My childhood years provoked many questions; I wanted to know why my mother was sick and suffered so much. The questions and the desire to understand have served me well throughout my life, as I have discovered so much about the human body and what it takes and the care that it needs to be strong and healthy.

INTESTINAL TRACT: DIGESTION AND IMMUNITY

How do man-made wheat proteins from modern bread and pasta damage our body? The key is understanding how they are digested.

Our intestinal tract is the first mechanism of defense for our immune system. The body first separates the toxins as they pass through the villi within the gut wall and the intestinal tract, which is fascinating when you think of the complexity of such a remarkable process.

The epithelial cells of the intestines are connected by structures called tight junctions. At the tip of these cells are the microvilli, which are like little microscopic vacuum hoses. As the villi are working and massaging the food to break it down, microvilli suck the particles up like little vacuum hoses, whether it's vitamin A or a pesticide from a carrot. The villi are not respecters of what they take. Their responsibility is to increase the absorption from the digestion of the nutrients and transport them through the epithelial cells into the bloodstream.

During the normal digestive process, these little tight junctions stay closed, forcing all of the molecules to effectively be screened and pass into the bloodstream only through the mucosal cells.

Since the villi are responsible for the screening process, these tight junctions fatigue under the constant bombardment of toxins such as hybrid gluten and chemicals. Once they fatigue, they start to loosen up, creating a more permeable condition that allows the unscreened molecules, or the larger undigested molecules, to flow directly into the bloodstream. It's like dipping a fishing net into a river and scooping up a big fish with little fish. You might capture the big one, but the little ones will go right through the holes and back into the water. This is called a leaky gut.

The leaky gut condition damages microvilli along the intestinal wall, so they cannot manufacture the digestive enzymes needed to break down the food, allowing food molecules to flow into the bloodstream freely, even those that have not been completely broken down into absorbable nutrients that your body needs.

The undigested foods and chemicals that are absorbed into the bloodstream now become your worst enemy. The strange proteins in hybridized wheat go right into your blood! The immune system naturally reacts because it doesn't know what else to do, and these food intolerances begin to unleash inflammation throughout the entire body.

Besides bread (think about that hybrid pizza crust), how many other of your favorite foods could be contributing to health issues?

Filtered Water

Drinking plenty of filtered water is also very important because it enhances the activity of the enzymes and natural flora in the gut, both of which work together to maintain GI health. This in turn facilitates better digestion, absorption, and utilization of the nutrients.

Live Enzymes

Foods that have live enzymes and that are not hybridized or genetically modified can improve gut health and deliver a high payload of nutrients without triggering inflammation and toxicity.

Food nutrients are dead when they are overcooked, microwaved, packaged, or canned years or months ago. They are dead when they are sprayed with pesticides, insecticides, and food preservatives to keep them looking good in the store or are gassed with carbon dioxide to stimulate ripening, in addition to being hybridized or genetically modified.

Pre- and Probiotics

Having a good amount of intestinal flora is important for us to have proper digestion and absorption. Stress, trauma, hospital stays for sickness or surgeries, drugs, antibiotics, and painkillers of any kind, sugars, and hybrid grains will compromise, if not destroy, the balance of natural intestinal flora and the integrity of the gut wall and the stomach mucosal lining. The entire GI tract needs to have a well-furbished supply of flora to activate and utilize the enzymes.

Probiotics are very essential for building the intestinal flora, maintaining good health, and fighting against the onset of gluten intolerance, celiac disease, or candida. The lack of intestinal flora weakens the body's ability to fight against the invasion of toxins that can be prevented by the presence of pre- and probiotics.

Increasing the good bacteria by taking pre- and probiotics will help establish proper flora in the GI tract and will inhibit the bad bacteria and overgrowth of yeast. Healing the gut lining helps with absorption of nutrients. Some studies suggest that keeping a ratio of 85 percent good to bad bacteria in the gut will stop the negative cycle from starting again.

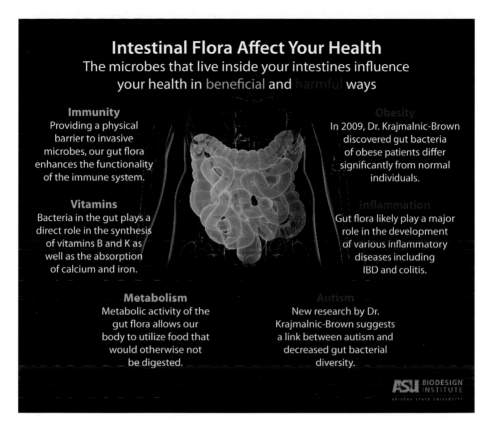

Intestinal Flora Affect Your Health
The microbes that live inside your intestines influence
your health in beneficial and harmful ways

Immunity
Providing a physical
barrier to invasive
microbes, our gut flora
enhances the functionality
of the immune system.

Vitamins
Bacteria in the gut plays a
direct role in the synthesis
of vitamins B and K as
well as the absorption
of calcium and iron.

Metabolism
Metabolic activity of the
gut flora allows our
body to utilize food that
would otherwise not
be digested.

Obesity
In 2009, Dr. Krajmalnic-Brown
discovered gut bacteria
of obese patients differ
significantly from normal
individuals.

Inflammation
Gut flora likely play a major
role in the development
of various inflammatory
diseases including
IBD and colitis.

Autism
New research by Dr.
Krajmalnic-Brown suggests
a link between autism and
decreased gut bacterial
diversity.

ASU BIODESIGN INSTITUTE
ARIZONA STATE UNIVERSITY

If you have a milk allergy with a low tolerance to lactose, you need a way to combat the body's inability to digest the milk. A good probiotic would help immensely. Most bacteria sold comes from pasteurized milk and has to first be cultured in the GI tract so that it can attach to the gut wall and continue culturing in order to be able to inhibit the bad bacteria.

The pasteurization process destroys the natural enzymatic activity that creates the fermentation for the lactobacillus to grow. Lactobacillus that has been pasteurized and/or radiated lacks the ability to attach to the GI wall and culture.

Perhaps you take three or four capsules or tablets to help, but then you eat and feel bloated or have diarrhea. This is because the lactobacillus bifidus that you took did not culture and only liquefied the food, causing diarrhea. Your health professional then tells you that you took too much when in reality, it just didn't culture and attach.

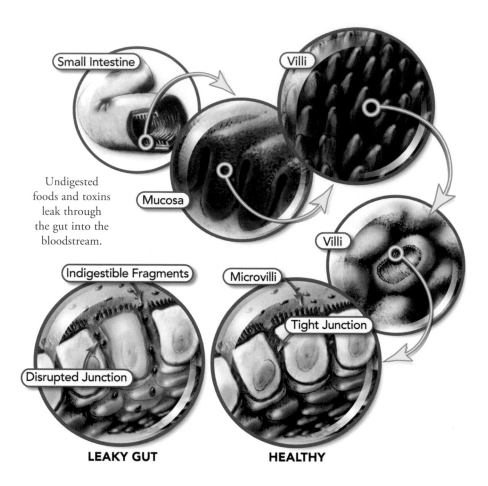

Small Intestine

Villi

Undigested
foods and toxins
leak through
the gut into the
bloodstream.

Mucosa

Villi

Indigestible Fragments

Microvilli

Tight Junction

Disrupted Junction

LEAKY GUT

HEALTHY

LEAKY GUT SYNDROME

Permeability of the gut wall, termed "leaky gut," permits toxins, bacteria, and undigested food proteins to seep through the gastrointestinal (GI) barrier and into the bloodstream. Research suggests that it is an early biological change that comes before the onset of multiple autoimmune diseases.

Several of the problems related to leaky gut syndrome are poorly digested foods and the overtaxing of the organs responsible for filtering the foods such as the spleen and liver. The lactose in those products can also create fermentation in the gut, leading to the toxins leaching into the blood vessels.

Once the toxins are in the blood vessels, this contributes to symptoms and the feeling of brain fatigue.

Many medical professionals debate the causes of leaky gut syndrome. Some say it is just a fad disease and really does not exist. But as soon as family members develop it, they hurry and go to the natural medical practitioner, who recognizes that it is very much a serious condition.

More research is being done, more articles are being published, more evidence is coming to the surface, and more and more mainstream doctors are starting to realize that they have been wrong.

Leaky gut syndrome is a condition that has been widely misunderstood until recently. What has yet to be proven is how much leaky gut syndrome is related to some of the other diseases.

Intestinal permeability is carefully regulated for a good reason. We now know that wheat gliadin triggers the release of the protein zonulin, which takes apart the tight junctions like a weight lifter wiping out a 90-pound weakling. Before we realize it, undigested food particles and proteins from the wheat slip through the junction holes into the bloodstream, triggering an inflammatory immune response. The gliadin and zonulin have caused unscreened molecules, including the larger undigested molecules, to flow *directly* into the bloodstream.

Now your gut is leaking! Your worst enemy is the undigested foods that are being absorbed into the bloodstream. Your immune system will naturally develop reactions to them because it doesn't know what else to do. Because of gut inflammation, the body produces gas and you feel bloated and more fatigued.

But there is more to just the food molecules escaping. The leaky gut allows the toxins, gases, acids, and yeast created from the lack of digestion to pass through the holes to flow freely into the bloodstream, causing fatigue, brain fog, headaches, memory loss, and a number of other problems.

Gliadin from modern hybrid wheat is **super inflammatory, super addictive, and super fattening.** It triggers systemic inflammation, leading to any number of autoimmune diseases like multiple sclerosis, chronic fatigue, fibromyalgia, irritable bowel syndrome, ulcerative colitis, and others.

Leaky gut syndrome is not a diagnosis taught in medical school. One gastroenterologist admitted that "Physicians don't know enough about the gut, which is our biggest immune system."[30]

The big questions remain, "Is it fixable and if so, how?" The medical community offers steroids and anti-inflammatories, which creates a hopeless situation. Some put their patients on restricted diets. Unfortunately, they restrict some of the foods that are critical to building their system and maintaining nutritional balance. This starts a cascading depletion of nutrients in the body that in perhaps weeks, months, or years will begin to manifest other symptoms related to immune compromise, nutritional compromise, and disease.

Remember: Modern hybrid wheat is **super inflammatory, super addictive, and super fattening.**

SCHIZOPHRENIA

According to PubMed Health:

Schizophrenia is a mental disorder that makes it hard to:

- Tell the difference between what is real and not real
- Think clearly
- Have normal emotional responses
- Act normally in social situations[31]

It has many symptoms from trouble concentrating and sleeping to problems paying attention and bizarre behaviors.

Through the years, studies have been conducted about the relationship between schizophrenia and gluten sensitivity that indicate that some relationship exists.

A study by the Karolinska Institutet in Sweden and Johns Hopkins Children's Center in the United States investigated links between maternal antibodies to gliadin and later diagnosis of psychiatric disorders in children born to such mothers.

A news release from the Institutet stated, "Babies born to women with sensitivity to gluten appear to be at increased risk of developing schizophrenia and other psychiatric disorders later in life. . . . The results of the study show that children born to mothers with abnormally high levels of antibodies to gliadin had nearly twice the risk of developing non-affective psychosis later in life, compared with children who had normal levels of gliadin antibodies.[32]

"There are studies in the past that show that people diagnosed with schizophrenia more often than others are suffering from various forms of immune responses to gluten. We will now conduct follow-up studies to clarify how gluten or sensitivity to it increases schizophrenia risk and whether it does so only in those genetically predisposed," said Dr. Karlsson,"[33] the lead researcher.

There is no scientific doubt that gluten can cause depression, anxiety, and even more serious mental disorders. A study done over 60 years ago found that the rates of schizophrenia during World War II went down as wheat was rationed in the generational population.[34]

In 1984 a study was performed showing only two cases of schizophrenia out of a population of 65,000 pre-westernized South Pacific residents who did not consume wheat products, but once westernized with a wheat, barley beer, and rice diet, they saw the rates climb to European levels.[35]

TOXIC TIME BOMB

We often forget to take into consideration all of the exposure to the radiation, radon, and other environmental toxins that we ingest with our food every day, let alone the direct poisons from sprays, fertilizers, and pesticides.

The process of digestion and the secretion of enzymes is complex and has a delicate balance. All of the toxins like pesticides, herbicides, and preservatives interact with the candida and the sugars to create a toxic time bomb in the gut. You feel fatigued and groggy after eating as the toxins start seeping into the bloodstream and cross the blood-brain barrier, compromising the function of the thyroid that slows down digestion. It is an ongoing circle of disaster that few people know how to change.

Why are diseases growing so rapidly throughout the world today? It all begins at the table.

Remember what Dr. Mark Hyman says: "The end of your fork is more powerful than the bottom of your pill bottle."[36]

ENDNOTES

1   Malkmus P, Malkmus A. GMO vs Hybrid: What's the Difference? *Health News Magazine.* http://www.hahealthnews.com/ampm/gmo-vs-hybrid-whats-the-difference/.

2   http://www.huffingtonpost.com/2013/06/05/monsanto-modified-wheat-oregon_n_3390825.html.

3   Ibid.

4   http://rt.com/usa/monsanto-gmo-wheat-crop-648/.

5   Hitti M. A Healthy Gut May Resist Allergies, Asthma. WebMed. 2/23/2004. http://www.webmd.com/allergies/news/20041223/healthy-gut-may-resist-allergies-asthma.

6   http://www.templegrandin.com/.

7   Ludvigsson JF, et al. A nationwide study of the association between celiac disease and the risk of autism spectrum disorders. *JAMA Psychiatry.* 2013 Nov;70(11):1224-30. http://www.autismspeaks.org/science/science-news/autism-study-finds-no-link-celiac-disease-gluten-reactivity-real.

8   Endo EH, Ueda-Nakamura T, Nakamura CV, Filho BP. Activity of spray-dried microparticles containing pomegranate peel extract against Candida albicans. *Molecules.* 2012 Aug 24;17(9):10094-107.

9   Bakkiyaraj D, Nandhini JR, Malathy B, Pandian SK. The anti-biofilm potential of pomegranate (Punica granatum L.) extract against human bacterial and fungal pathogens. *Biofouling.* 2013 Sep;29(8):929-37.

10 McCombs, J. Connecting Gluten Allergies and Candida Albicans. 9/10/2011. http://www.healthiertalk.com/connecting-gluten-allergies-and-candida-albicans-4644.

11 http://www.naturalnews.com/036845_wheat_belly_weight_gain_gluten.html.

12 Lapid N. How Common is Celiac Disease? Celiac Disease & Gluten Sensitivity. About.com. Updated April 17, 2014. http://celiacdisease.about.com/od/faqs/f/HowCommon.htm.

13 http://www.mayo.edu/research/discoverys-edge/celiac-disease-rise.

14 Ibid.

15 Rubio-Tapia A, Kyle RA, Kaplan EL, et al. Increased prevalence and mortality in undiagnosed celiac disease. *Gastroenterology.* 2009 Jul;137(1):88-93.

16 Lohi S, Mustalahti K, Kaukinen K, et al. Increasing prevalence of coelic disease over time. *Ailment Pharmacol Ther.* 2007 Nov 1;26(9):1217-25.

17 Davis W, MD, *Wheat Belly,* Rodale, 2011:34.

18 http://www.huffingtonpost.com/dr-mark-hyman/wheat-gluten_b_1274872.html.

19 http://mednews.com/seniors-dementia-statistics.

20 http://www.fightdementia.org.au/understanding-dementia/statistics.aspx.

21 Fawcett E. Could Eating Gluten Cause Dementia Symptoms and Alzheimer's? *Natural Health Advisory Daily;* 6/20/2012. http://www.naturalhealthadvisory.com/daily/cognitive-decline-and-memory-issues/could-eating-gluten-cause-dementia-symptoms-and-alzheimer%e2%80%99s/.

22 Elvidge S, BSc (hons), MSc. Statistics: How Many People Have FMS. Updated 26 January 2013. http://www.fibromyalgiasyndrome.co.uk/how-many-people-have-fms.html.

23 Fibromyalgia Health Center. WebMed. http://www.webmd.com/fibromyalgia/guide/what-is-fibromyalgia.

24 http://www.huffingtonpost.com/dr-mark-hyman/wheat-gluten_b_1274872.html.

25 Ibid.

26 Davis W, MD, *Wheat Belly,* Rodale, 2011:26.

27 Johannsen NM, et al. Association of white blood cells subfraction concentration with fitness and fatness. *Br J Sports Med.* 2010 Jun;44(8):588-93.

28 Imayaja I, et al. Effects of a caloric restriction weight loss diet and exercise on inflammatory biomarkers in overweight/obese postmenopausal women: a randomized controlled trial. *Cancer Res.* 2012 May 1;72(9):2314-26.

29 Assimes T. Large-scale association analysis identifies new risk loci for coronary artery disease. *Nat Gen.* 2013 Jan;45(1):25-33.

30 http://www.webmd.com/digestive-disorders/features/leaky-gut-syndrome.

31 http://www.ncbi.nlm.nih.gov/pubmedhealth/PMH0001925/.

32 Karlsson H, Blomström A, Wicks S, Yang S, Yolken RH, Dalman C. Maternal Antibodies to Dietary Antigens and Risk for Nonaffective Psychosis in Offspring. *Am J Psychiatry*, Epub ahead of print. 25 April 2012. http://ki.se/en/news/maternal-gluten-sensitivity-linked-to-schizophrenia-risk-in-children.

33 Ibid.

34 Dohan FC. Wheat "consumption" and hospital admissions for schizophrenia during World War II. A preliminary report. *Am J Clin Nutr.* 1966 Jan;18(1):7-10.

35 Dohan FC, et al. Is schizophrenia rare if grain is rare? *Biol Psychiatry.* 1984 Mar;19(3):385-99.

36 http://www.huffingtonpost.com/dr-mark-hyman/wheat-gluten_b_1274872.html.

CHAPTER 7

The Silent Killers the Pharmaceutical Companies Love

f you are an average American adult, especially if you are a senior citizen, research shows that your body is polluted with approximately 700 synthetic chemicals and heavy metals like mercury, lead, and arsenic. The fact is, we are bombarded constantly by pollutants that come from a wide variety of sources, including, but not limited to, household cleaning detergents, pesticides, canned foods, recirculated airline air, prescription and over-the-counter drugs, and even personal-care products. Yes, even products used every day such as shampoos, deodorants, aftershave, lipsticks, makeup, and antibacterial soaps contain hundreds of synthetic chemicals and toxins that can harm your health in a major way.

Many people have used different traditional detoxification methods to reduce the toxins in their body, which for some has been shocking to see the effect of making the body more toxic. The good news is that breakthroughs in nutritional medicine now make it possible to eliminate these toxins more efficiently than has ever before been accomplished.

Our "toxic burden" is something we don't like to think about. We are heavily laden with toxic chemicals that don't belong in our body, including PCBs, dioxins, plasticizers, heavy metals such as mercury, cadmium, and lead. Avoidance is always the best way to protect yourself. Our environment is polluted with so many toxins that all of us are affected. Over 80,000 POPs— persistent organic pollutants—have been released into the

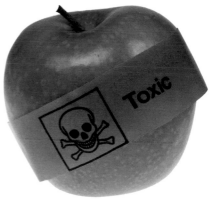

environment. Unfortunately, we lack information on how many of these affect human health. Therefore, detoxification is an essential part of maintaining health in the 21st century.

We do not understand the total effects these toxins have on the human body. Many of the toxins we deal with are causing cancer. They disrupt or weaken our immune system by creating inflammation in the gastrointestinal tract. Many of them cause birth defects, hormonal disruption, and infertility. Neurotoxins are creating mental disorders and neurological behavior dysfunctions. These are health repercussions because of neurotoxins and poisons such as lead, PCBs, mercury, and thimerosol (found in some vaccines). These toxins can cause a long list of serious health conditions and may even act as precursors to many of today's modern neurological diseases. Mounting evidence shows that many of the diseases and illnesses that plague mankind today may be directly or indirectly linked to toxicity.

What is happening? Our liver, spleen, and lungs—our major filtration organs—are over-polluted; and we do very little to facilitate servicing our body. In contrast, we are careful about servicing our car. We have the oil changed, the tires rotated, the engine checked when we think there might be a problem, the windshield repaired or replaced when it's chipped or cracked; and we make sure we use the right kind of fuel.

We often take better care of our automobile than we do of our body; yet whenever there's a malfunction in our body, we ask what happened. We don't look at the fact that our "engine" wasn't designed to function well on the hybrid grains, GMO foods, sweeteners, artificial colorings, additives, preservatives, chemicals, and other toxins we put into our "tank."

If all human beings would learn to service their body as they service their car, clean it out, make sure they eat the best quality of food to get a "high octane" response, and avoid the "low octane" foods that will cause misfiring in the body like it would cause misfiring in an engine, we would see greater performance, longer life, and much happier outcomes.

We are exposed to so many toxins that the liver and the rest of the body can't handle the elimination of all of them as fast as we are bombarded with them. This will cause inflammation in the liver and in the gallbladder, which generally results in gallstones. It inhibits the secretion from the gallbladder and can inhibit the secretion of bile into the digestive tract for the facilitation of the breakdown of proteins, starches, and fats. In addition, it doesn't enable the liver to cleanse itself. The liver is responsible for carrying out over 3,000 chemical functions in the body daily. A congested liver will contribute to diseases, nutritional deficiencies, and cancer.

We unintentionally produce chemicals such as dioxins as a result of industrial processes from combustion, municipal and medical waste incineration, and backyard trash burning.

It has been said that agriculture alone, which takes up 37 percent of the non-ice landmass around the world, produces more toxins than all industries combined. Why? Because of the factories that produce fertilizers, pesticides, herbicides, and sprays. In addition, the methane from pigs, sheep, cows, and goats all goes into the atmosphere, and chemicals leach into the aquifer from the commercial farms.

Foods are sprayed with pesticides and fertilizers. Some people say we need to just *wash* our fruits and vegetables. Will that help? Yes, it will help. But does it get rid of them? No. Once the fruits and vegetables are sprayed, the pesticide goes into the skin. It will even penetrate into the core. It has been found that three times more chemicals sprayed on apples is found in the core than on the peeling of the apple. So if the chemicals go completely through the apple to the core, how likely is it that washing will get rid of them?

These pollutants decrease both the conversion and the production of the thyroid hormone, just as chlorine blocks the uptake of tyrosine in the thyroid and TSH from the anterior pituitary. Alarmingly, bathing in a tub of chlorine for 20 minutes is equivalent to drinking eight glasses of chlorinated water.

Toxic compounds have also been shown to interfere with the action of the thyroid hormone that helps give us energy. Even if you have the right amount of active T3, toxins may prevent T3 and T4 from doing their jobs. This can result in symptoms of hypothyroidism, despite perfect thyroid levels.

Toxins are fat soluble, which means they dissolve in fat and oil, not water. That's why they are stored in the fat cells in your body. Your liver is the largest fat-storing organ in the body, so it can contain up to 200 times more chemicals than your blood. Toxins stored in fat are relatively stable and contained, but once you lose weight or start a traditional detox program, the toxins will dump out of the fat cells and go straight into the bloodstream. Toxins circulating in your blood can reach your vital organs, wreaking havoc on your health, not to mention invading your joints, tissues, brain, heart, endocrine system, pancreas, eyes, and stomach.

Once unleashed into your bloodstream by traditional types of detoxing, the side effects of toxins being released increase pain, inflammation, headaches, memory loss, premature brain aging, brain fatigue, brain fog, blood pressure problems, estrogen dominance, sexual dysfunction, blood sugar imbalance, vision problems, nausea, vomiting, neurological dysfunction, and behavioral problems.

Therefore, a person who is losing weight needs to go through a detoxification program to eliminate the toxins that are being dumped into the blood stream.

THE SILENT KILLERS

Many food additives, enhancers, artificial flavors, stabilizers, preservatives, and colorings are used in our food today. Fast foods, snacks, sweets, and desserts, the whole food chain, have been invaded with what are called the "silent killers." These additives are contributing factors to conditions we refer to as irritable bowel syndrome, Crohn's disease, diverticulitis, food sensitivities, gluten intolerance, and celiac disease.

This bombardment is in our food, atmosphere, and water—in everything. According to the Pew Health Initiative[1] there are "more than 10,000 additives allowed in food" that we deal with daily, not to mention over 700 different chemicals from PCBs to POPs, which are persistent organic pollutants. Many pollutants are airborne, and others come through our food chain, water supply, and that which we put on topically.

The diseases with fancy names for which the pharmaceutical companies have created drugs and from which people are having side effects come down to pretty much the same thing—we have destroyed our gastrointestinal tracts because our gut is not able to recognize these synthetics and does not know which enzymes to secrete to combat them. We no longer have an adequate supply of enzymes in our gut because of the way we have lived throughout the last couple of decades. This has greatly compromised the enzymes in our body.

Being enzyme deficient makes it even more of a challenge for our body to break down the man-made substances. Just look at what our bodies have to contend with daily.

ARTIFICIAL COLORS

Artificial colors can cause allergic reactions and hyperactivity,
and there have been some links to cancer. Even natural
ingredients may contain artificial colors.

Each color has very specific details.

- **Blue No. 1**, found in baking goods, beverages, dessert powders, candies, cereals, etc., may have caused kidney tumors in mice.
- **Blue No. 2** is found in colored beverages, candy, and other foods and has caused brain tumors in male rats. Blue Nos. 1 and 2 are used in the coloring of gel capsules used in some natural health food products, so when you find a health food company that puts out products in blue capsules, beware.
- **Citrus Red No. 2** is sprayed on some green Florida oranges to make them look ripe. It can cause cancer if the peel is eaten.
- **Green No. 3** is found in drugs, personal-care items, cosmetic products (but none for the eye area), candies, beverages, puddings, ice cream, sherbet, cherries, baked goods, and dairy products. It caused increases in bladder and testes tumors in male rats.
- **Red No. 3** was recognized by the FDA as a thyroid carcinogen in animals and is banned in cosmetics and externally applied drugs. It's in sausage casing, oral medication, maraschino cherries, baked goods, and candies.
- **Red No. 40** is perhaps the most widely used artificial color and is used in soda pop, gelatin desserts, pastries, and condiments and is a suspected carcinogen.
- Yellow No. 5 is the second most widely used color and contributes to behavioral disturbances in children. It is being tested for links to hyperactivity, anxiety, migraines, and cancer. Reactions to it are primarily found in aspirin-sensitive individuals. It is found in gelatin, pet foods, desserts, candy, baked goods, pharmaceutical drugs, and cosmetics.
- Yellow No. 6 has caused animal adrenal tumors and can cause severe hypersensitivity reactions. It is found in beverages, sausage, colored baked goods, candy, gelatin, cosmetics, and drugs.

Artificial Sweeteners

Artificial sweeteners are chemicals that exist to make our food sweeter and help prevent weight gain. Artificial sweeteners are supposed to reduce calories while allowing us our treats, but the amazing thing is that our nation has been getting fatter since the widespread introduction of these artificial sweeteners in our food supply. Why? What is wrong? What are the dangers of artificial sweeteners?

When we eat something sweet that does not contain any calories, our body feels deprived and craves *more* calories, so we keep eating.

What are these sweeteners made of? They're derived from petrochemicals. Some of these petrochemicals have a half-life in the tissue of the body for over 12 years.

These artificial substances are very acidic, and acid creates inflammation. Inflammation takes oxygen out of the tissues. This causes pain and is a host for the onset and development of future diseases.

We've created this endless cycle from these artificial sweeteners, where many people continue to eat, gain more weight, and have cravings for more sweet foods. The sweeteners are truly addictive.

Also, most of the foods that contain artificial sweeteners have very little or no nutritional value. In a sense, our body is starved no matter how much we eat. We are still hungry all of the time because our body is not getting the nutrients it needs to satisfy it.

Most of these artificial sweeteners have side effects that we are not even aware of; and often when we have a side effect, we blame it on something else.

Our acids and enzymes try to break them down and digest these man-made molecules and in process create toxic intermediates. These in combination with other food additives like colorings, synthetic preservatives, stabilizers, synthetic extenders, or flavoring agents like MSG create a chemical soup that is not conducive to health.

What are these chemicals doing to our bodies?

A 2006 study from the University of Liverpool found that two chemical combinations that any child might encounter from a snack and a soda had synergistic negative effects, killing neurons in mouse neuroblastoma (brain) cells. The two combinations included blue food coloring and L-glutamic acid (aka MSG), and yellow food coloring and aspartame. All of these artificial colors, flavors, and sweeteners are bad enough on their own, but now there is proof that when they combine, they are even more hazardous.[2]

Aspartame. Aspartame is the synthetic sweetener that is marketed under different names. The scary part is that people with diabetes who are not aware of its problems may use aspartame instead of table sugar. You will find it in sugar-free beverages, gums, candies, instant and low-calorie desserts, drink mixes, gelatins, diet sodas, power bars, drinks, and even chewable vitamins for children. It is in thousands of different food and drink products. It is even in health products. If desserts are sugar-free, they will often be sweetened with aspartame.

The side effects of aspartame and all other artificial sweeteners may be insomnia, ringing in the ears, hallucinations, dizziness, seizures, blurred vision, rashes, depression, headaches, muscle spasms, weight gain, fatigue, irritability, tachycardia, hearing loss, heart palpitations, anxiety attacks, slurred speech, loss of appetite, tendonitis, vertigo, memory loss, and joint pain.

Dr. Janet Hull, who has a doctorate in nutrition, studied the adverse effects of aspartame; and in her book, *Sweet Poison,*[3] she lists the following chronic illnesses that can be triggered or worsened by ingesting aspartame: brain tumors, multiple sclerosis, epilepsy, chronic fatigue syndrome, Parkinson's, Alzheimer's, mental retardation, lymphoma, birth defects, fibromyalgia, and diabetes.

Saccharin. The sweetener saccharin has a controversial safety record, based on findings of bladder cancer in male rats fed sodium saccharin in the late '70s. It is still used in some products and in 1997 was required to carry a warning as a carcinogen, but in 2000 the warning was dropped. Does that make it safe? Look at the money behind it and what the real objective is of pushing products that contain saccharin.

Consume those sweeteners and you will get a tasty helping of chlorine atoms, benzoic sulfilimine, and aspartame. Aspartame is made of methanol, phenylalanine, and aspartic acid. Methanol (methyl alcohol) can be converted to formaldehyde in such sensitive areas of the body as your brain. These chemicals alter brain neurochemistry.

People argue that phenylalanine is an amino acid. It is, but in this case it's a *synthetic* amino. Synthetic phenylalanine is very sweet but poorly absorbed by the body.

Sucralose. The most recent sweeteners to hit the market contain sucralose and are synthetic chemicals that are made by chemically reacting sucrose with chlorine. Chlorine blocks the uptake of tyrosine and iodine for the thyroid.

No long-term human toxicity studies were done until *after* sucralose was approved for consumption. Then there was a study that lasted a whole three months, and *no* studies were ever done on children or pregnant women.

Tagatose. Although similar in texture to sucrose, tagatose is poorly absorbed by the body. It is about as "healthy" as sucralose.

Neotame. Similar to aspartame, neotame is considered more stable but still has all of the side effects that aspartame has.

Acesulfame-K. Acesulfame potassium has been around since 1967 as a calorie-free artificial sweetener. It is many times sweeter than table sugar, but it has a slightly bitter aftertaste. It is used in chewing gum, baked goods, and gelatin desserts. However, studies have shown that it may cause lung cancer and thymus gland tumors in animals. It is also linked to leukemia, chronic respiratory disease, and breast cancer in humans.

AZODICARBONAMIDE

The Environmental Working Group says that this chemical is in close to 500 food products.[4] **Even more troublesome, it has been embedded in the food supply** for quite some time and is found in most cereals and breads and also is used in the forming of plastic mats, rubber-soled shoes, yoga mats, and many other rubber products. It's even used in leathers, particularly in man-made leathers.

This chemical is allowed in bread products up to 45 ppm (parts per million). Why is it still legal in foods in the U.S. when it has been banned in Europe, Australia, and the United Kingdom? Again, we have to ask what the ulterior motive is of the regulatory agency that will allow these chemicals to be put into our food.

Natasha Longo, who has a master's degree in nutrition, explains how it is made and then explains its dangers:

This chemical is manufactured by the reaction of hydrazine sulfate and urea under high temperature and pressure. The product of this reaction is then oxidized using sodium chloride and centrifuged to yield a slurry containing azodicarbonamide. The slurry is washed to remove impurities and dried to obtain the chemical powder. This is then micronized to a fine powder before packaging and being put into your food chain.

Azodicarbonamide is used in the production of foam plastics like the gaskets around windows, shoe soles, and exercise mats. A chemically identical food-grade version is used to make your breads and cereals.

- In experimental mammals demonstrates acute toxicity
- Found to be a mutagen in bacterial systems
- Found to cause asthma and skin sensitization in humans
- Has killed dogs in experiments
- Banned in Europe and Australia and the United Kingdom

But it's okay to add as dough conditioners & bleaching agents to our breads and cereals to preserve shelf life?[5]

A number of websites ran an article to make us feel safe about this chemical: "How Dangerous is this . . . Bread Chemical? Those of you who bought a . . . sandwich for lunch probably don't need to worry, according to a 1999 World Health Organization evaluation. Studies on the effects of the chemical azodicarbonamide showed a negligible impact from the chemical in animal test subjects, except in massive doses. All information regarding human testing was inconclusive."[6]

What they failed to say about the animal testing is that the intestinal tract of the rat is not the same as that of a human. The absorption capacity is different, and the rat doesn't have a gallbladder that will break it down and make it more readily absorbable. So who do you believe? However, it just so happens that this one strange chemical is in two of the most addictive foods we have—breads and cereals.

GENETICALLY MODIFIED FOODS

Here is another part of the terrible future for the world's food supply— GMO (Genetically Modified Organism) foods. Today we have GMO corn, soybean, papayas, cotton, zucchini, yellow squash, canola, and other crops, as well as GMO crops that are used to produce dairy products and processed foods.

A Colorado State University fact sheet reported this: "The most common GE [genetically engineered] crops in the United States are soybean, corn, cotton, and canola. Because many processed food products contain soybean or corn ingredients (e.g., high fructose corn syrup or soy protein), it's estimated that

60 to 70 percent of processed foods in grocery stores include at least one GE ingredient."[7]

LiveStrong health writer Janine Grant reports:

> You most likely eat at least some GMOs. Crops that are genetically modified to resist herbicides or produce insecticides came on the market in 1996. According to the Organic Consumers Association, 40 percent of all U.S. crops are GMO, and 80 percent of processed foods contain GMOs. GMO crops are also used as a cheap and fattening feed for factory-farmed animals, which are also often injected with genetically engineered hormones. The USDA reports that 88 percent of corn and 93 percent of soybeans are GMOs, as are 90 percent of cotton and canola.[8]

The most disturbing aspect to GMO is that there seems to be no mandatory safety testing, and thus there is no clear proof that these foods are safe. Was a long-term safety study done on GMO corn? The French researcher Gilles-Eric Séralini did in 2009.

Mike Adams of *Natural News* wrote about this study that caused Europe to rethink GMO foods:

- Up to 50% of males and 70% of females suffered premature death.
- Rats that drank trace amounts of [glyphosate] (at levels legally allowed in the water supply) had a 200% to 300% increase in large tumors.
- Rats fed GMO corn and traces of [glyphosate] suffered severe organ damage, including liver damage and kidney damage.
- The study fed these rats NK6023, the . . . variety of GMO corn that's

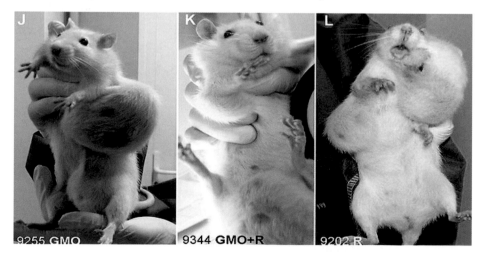

grown across North America and widely fed to animals and humans. This is the same corn that's in your corn-based breakfast cereal, corn tortillas and corn snack chips.[9]

Séralini conducted an even longer study in 2012, where he studied rats fed [glyphosate]-tolerant genetically modified corn for two years. The study reports:

In females, all treated groups died 2-3 times more than controls, and more rapidly. This difference was visible in 3 male groups fed GMOs. . . . Females developed large mammary tumors almost always more often than and before controls, the pituitary was the second most disabled organ. . . . In treated males, liver congestions and necrosis were 2.5–5.5 time higher. . . . Males presented 4 times more large palpable tumors than controls which occurred up to 600 days earlier.[10]

GMO foods will increase food toxicity, allergic systems, weakened immune systems, resistance to antibiotics, and the incidence of cancer, which has been proven in laboratory animals fed GMO foods, as you can see above.[11]

MSG

MSG, monosodium glutamate, is a very popular flavoring agent and is used as a flavor enhancer to give foods a richer flavor. A lot of popular Oriental and Mexican foods that we like so much contain MSG, which is a very toxic substance.

MSG was developed in 1908 by processing glutamic acid from seaweed. The original process was slow and costly. According to the organization Truth in Labeling, by 1956 the Ajinomoto Co., Inc. found a less expensive method to produce glutamic acid by fermentation. The process is "a method of bacterial fermentation wherein bacteria (some, if not all of which are genetically modified) are grown aerobically in a liquid nutrient medium. These bacteria have the ability to synthesize glutamic acid outside of their cell membranes and excrete it into the medium to accumulate there."[12]

Not exactly tasty. We are told that glutamic acid is a natural amino acid found in protein and created in the body when needed. What we aren't told is that the processed glutamic acid is *not* the same as what is found naturally in proteins or created in the body and that all processed glutamic acid comes with impurities; this does not happen in the natural protein version or what is created by the body.

You may be familiar with chirality. It's about "handedness," where your left hand is the mirror image of your right hand. But you cannot put a leather glove for the left hand on the right hand! They are opposites! Glutamic acid (the natural one) is like that. It has an L form (L-glutamic acid). The processed version contains some L-glutamic acid, but according to Truth in Labeling, there is more: "In addition to the inevitable production of D-glutamic acid (the mirror opposite of L-glutamic acid), impurities may include, but are not limited to, pyroglutamic acid, mono and dichloro propanols, and heterocyclic amines. Mono and dichloro propanols and heterocyclic amines are carcinogenic."[13]

MSG was written about in the classic 1996 book by Russell L. Blaylock, MD, called *Excitotoxins: The Taste That Kills*.[14] In his book he explains how the dangers of MSG were discovered.

In 1957 two ophthalmologists did animal research for an eye disorder. They fed MSG to newborn mice and found widespread destruction of an inner layer of the retina. In testing adult mice, there was similar destruction; but it was more severe in the newborn mice. Ten years before this 1957 study, large amounts of MSG were added to baby food, as Dr. Blaylock says, "in doses equal to those of the experimental animals."[15] The report was published and forgotten.

But in 1969, Dr. John Olney, a medical doctor and professor of psychiatry, pathology, and immunology at Washington University School of Medicine, repeated the early study and showed that lab animals suffered brain lesions and neuroendocrine disorders when exposed to monosodium glutamate. Dr. Olney also reported that the animals treated with monosodium glutamate became obese.[16]

Dr. Olney coined the term "excitotoxicity" to explain how glutamate can kill neurons by "exciting" them to death. His theory was not only rejected, but it was also ridiculed; and it took about 15 years before it became credible—to some. Dr. Olney is now the author of 142 peer-reviewed studies.

Industry sources say that glutamate cannot enter the brain to cause this damage because of the Blood Brain Barrier. But that does not appear to be true.

In his book Dr. Blaylock states, "It has also been demonstrated that high concentrations of blood glutamate and aspartate (from foods) can enter the so-called 'protected brain' by seeping through the unprotected areas, such as the hypothalamus or other circumventricular organs."[17]

There is a big campaign to quiet everyone down about MSG, which was grandfathered into the regulations as "generally regarded as safe" (GRAS), even though there has apparently never been any safety testing.

The Federation of American Societies for Experimental Biology (FASEB) published a 350-page report completed on July 31, 1995. The executive summary consists of responses to 18 questions. Few bother to find the entire report, which Dr. Blaylock has a lot to say about:

> The [agency] wrote a very deceptive summary of the report in which they implied that, except possibly for asthma patients, MSG was found to be safe by the FASEB reviewers. But, in fact, that is not what the report said at all. I summarized, in detail, my criticism of this widely reported . . . deception in the revised paperback edition of my book, *Excitotoxins: The Taste That Kills*, by analyzing exactly what the report said, and failed to say. For example, it never said that MSG did not aggravate neurodegenerative diseases. What they said was, there were no studies indicating such a link. Specifically, that no one has conducted any studies, positive or negative, to see if there is a link. A vital difference.[18]

The FASEB report does discuss the symptoms of "MSG Syndrome Complex" (previously called "Chinese Restaurant Syndrome"). It lists the following symptoms: burning sensation on back of neck and forearms; chest pain; headache; nausea; palpitations; numbness in back of neck radiating to arms and back; tingling, warmth, weakness in face, temples, upper back, neck, and arms; bronchospasm (observed in asthmatics only); drowsiness; weakness.[19]

People are now trying to avoid this excitotoxin. MSG, as such, has to be listed on food labels, but there are ways to get around that. There are over 40 ingredients that contain glutamic acid that you may not realize do *exactly* what MSG does, including autolyzed yeast, glutamate, calcium caseinate, gelatin, glutamic acid, hydrolyzed protein, monopotassium glutamate, monosodium glutamate, yeast extract, textured protein, gelatin, hydrolyzed protein, sodium caseinate, yeast food, and yeast nutrient. And then there is yet another list of ingredients that often contain MSG or create MSG during processing. Dr. Joseph Mercola has an article that is helpful.[20]

There was a strong political lobby in the early days concerning tobacco production and promotion. All involved in the tobacco industry assured the public that the consumption of tobacco would not have any adverse impact on health. The manufacturers, advertisers, and tobacco lobby had much at stake; but the truth about tobacco finally came out. Today's equivalent of tobacco is MSG, so it doesn't surprise us that the MSG alliance of the organizations attempting to ensure the ongoing sale of it keep promoting and defending MSG sales. It is shrouded by a cloak of deception and lies.

Many snack foods contain MSG as a flavoring and enhancer; be sure to read the labels.

Additives like MSG are making people sick. We are continually bombarded throughout the world today by chemicals, poisons, and toxins. Virtually everything we eat or drink reduces our quality of health.

PESTICIDES

Even the EPA says that "Laboratory studies show that pesticides can cause health problems, such as birth defects, nerve damage, cancer, and other effects that might occur over a long period of time."[21]

Each year more than 2 billion pounds of pesticides are applied to our food supply. That's about 10 pounds per person per year. And we wonder why we've got gut problems?

Cornell University reported on pesticide regulations stating that agencies can require up to 70 different kinds of specific tests that can cause manufacturers many millions of dollars. So why can you find hundreds of pesticide studies showing damage to human fertility? Nine years of tests? What kinds of tests?

Pesticides are found in our food supply. They pollute our water and the cells in our body. They are sprayed on our food crops, in our gardens, in our parks, and on playing fields. They are used on grass fields in the schools to kill the weeds and keep the fields looking green. What about the golf courses that people

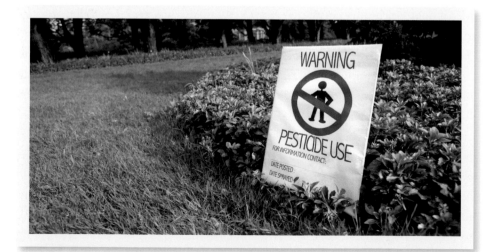

are walking on? As feet are walking, running, and sliding through it, the grass is disturbed and the pesticide will flash off because it has a gaseous residue. Why? It's made from petrochemicals. These pesticides accumulate in our body.

A study of breast milk from both a rural and an urban area of northern California found that of 24 chemicals tested, 13 were detected in 90 percent of the tests. Those chemicals included pesticides like chlorpyrifos, permethhrin, and PCBs.[22]

- DDT (dichlorodiphenyltrichloroethane) is a highly effective contact poison and was used extensively in agriculture as a pesticide in the mid-1900s. It has been linked to cancer, diabetes, and problems in the human reproductive system. It is also toxic to wildlife, especially birds and fish. Its use is now banned in most developed countries, but the effects of its prolonged, substantial use are yet to be completely known.

- All of us have measurable levels of polychlorinate biphenyls, PCBs. Why? We don't ingest it. But even though the manufacturing of PCBs was banned in the U.S. in 1979, they are still all around us in the environment.

- We have dioxin heptachlor, chlordane, aldrin, dieldrin, and other pesticides in our bloodstream. Where are they coming from? What chance do we have of having a toxin free body?

Fat soluble chemicals and toxins are dispersed into the bloodstream and stored in fat tissues, and weight loss can release them back into the body, according to a study by the CDC's National Health and Nutrition Examination Survey (NHANES). More than 1,000 people over the age of 40 were tested after weight loss, and six pollutants were identified in the blood.[23] What was *not* studied was if those released toxins from weight loss had any effects on health.

Since our weight often fluctuates, these toxins can weaken our endocrine system, wreaking havoc with our reproductive, circulatory, immune, and central nervous systems, not to mention that while these chemicals are circulating through our bloodstream, because they are all acidic agents, they create acidosis.

The likelihood of having heart disease, cancer, and of course allergies, which are indicators that our bodies are in trouble, has greatly increased in the last three decades.

Studies indicate that these pesticides without question impair fertility. The impact of 15 most used pesticides on male reproduction showed that pesticide exposure damages spermatozoa.[24]

Another study reported that "exposure to some pesticides can interfere with all developmental stages of reproductive function in adult females, including puberty, menstruation and ovulation, fertility and fecundity, and menopause."[25] Pesticides may also contribute to birth defects, miscarriages, and spontaneous abortions. We wonder why in America so many fertility clinics are opening today. We wonder why many of our young people, male and female, are sterile and cannot reproduce.

METHYLPHENIDATE/ATOMOXETINE

The claim to fame for methylphenidate is that it calms hyperactive children. Prescriptions are soaring. But experts warn of serious side effects, and it's even being linked to suicide, according to a British article published May 7, 2012.

In this 2012 article[26] by John Naish, he tells about one British mom who is happy her 10-year-old son can take a break during holidays, not only from his schoolwork but from the methylphenidate pills he takes every day for his ADHD. She says the drug dulls his hyperactive tendencies, but she wants him off the pills whenever possible. "When he is off [methylphenidate], he will run around, ride his bike, not sit still," she says. "But he sleeps and eats better. The drugs keep him wakeful and reduce his appetite."

Naish writes:

Andrea's reluctance to medicate her son's behavior unnecessarily seems very wise.

It showed that prescriptions of [methylphenidate] have quadrupled in the last decade, from 150,000 in 1999 to 661,463 in 2010, with children as young as three taking the powerful medication. This massive growth comes despite warnings from experts that the more children take ADHD drugs, the more 'rare' but lethal side-effects such as suicidal thoughts and psychosis become common.

This human toll was starkly revealed at the inquest last year of 10-year-old Harry Hucknall, who killed himself while on a high dose of [methylphenidate]. The youngster . . . had ADHD. The level of [methylphenidate] found in his system was above the normal therapeutic level, and he was also on drugs for depression when he was found at his home in Dalton, September 2010. The West Cumbria coroner, Ian Smith, said doctors must be "extremely careful" in prescribing drugs to 10-year-olds. "We as a society should stop dabbling in street drugs, and yet a child with the label of ADHD is prescribed mind-altering drugs of a very powerful nature, the full consequence of which I do not believe we fully understand or are prepared to deal with."

The case echoes an earlier tragedy, in 2008, when 15-year-old Anthony Cole hanged himself in his bedroom after his [methylphenidate] prescription was increased. The Milton Keynes schoolboy had been on the drug for six years, having been diagnosed with ADHD at the age of nine.[27]

In this article, it states that the British Association of Educational Psychologists were seeing a worrying new trend, "its members are seeing [methylphenidate] dosages being increased over time."

John Naish then tells how Dave Traxson, an educational psychologist, states that psychiatrists are ignoring their own guidelines:

. . . which stress that children who show evidence of anxiety should not be put on [methylphenidate]-type stimulant drugs. Children who are anxious may misbehave and be fidgety, but those symptoms must not be mistaken as ADHD. . . . The last thing you want if you're feeling anxious is to take a stimulant drug. The guidelines also advise that children on these drugs be weighed every six months, as the medication can severely shrink their appetite. This rule is being breached all over the country. One group of psychiatrists told me point blank that they do not have the staff to do this. If they haven't the resources to do the thing safely, should they be doing it at all?[28]

Peter Kinderman, Professor of Clinical Psychology at the University of Liverpool, is quoted in Naish's article saying: "Children are being prescribed medication as a quick fix, rather than being given full assessment and psychological therapies, which may take longer and cost more, but ultimately are better in the long run."

John Naish concludes, "Indeed, recent research proves that drug-free approaches can dispel the symptoms of ADHD."

Let's state that again! "**Indeed, recent research proves that drug-free approaches can dispel the symptoms of ADHD.**"[29] [Emphasis added]

The University of Colorado conducted a study that was published in 2010 where 70 teens (13 to 19 years old) who were diagnosed with ADHD and also had substance abuse disorder were randomly assigned to receive cognitive behavioral therapy and either atomoxetine or a placebo for 12 weeks. The results? Both groups had a decrease in ADHD symptoms, and there was **no difference** between the drug group and the placebo group.[30]

There is a big promotion for atomoxetine. It is considered a non-stimulant that may provide relief for ADHD symptoms. The promotion on this drug says it is approved for the treatment of Attention Deficit Hyperactive Disorder, ADHD, in children age 6 and older, teens, and adults. This drug should be used as part of a total treatment program for ADHD that may include counseling or other therapies."[31]

However, here is the rest:

What is the most important information I should know about [atomoxetine]? Suicidal thoughts and actions in children and teenagers.

Children and teenagers sometimes think about suicide, and many report trying to kill themselves. In some children and teens, [atomoxetine] increases the risk of suicidal thoughts or actions. Results from [atomoxetine's] clinical studies with over 2200 children or teenage ADHD patients suggest that some children and teenagers may have a higher chance of having suicidal thoughts or actions. Although no suicides occurred in these studies, 4 out of every 1000 patients developed suicidal thoughts. Call the doctor right away if your child or teenager has thoughts of suicide or sudden changes in mood or behavior, especially at the beginning of the treatment or after a change in dosage. [Atomoxetine] is not approved for major depressive disorder.[32]

Let's look at an earlier review of ADHD studies by Dr. A. Daniel Waschbusch of the University of Buffalo-SUNY, who found the placebo effect not in the children receiving medication in studies but in the parents and teachers of those students.

Dr. Waschbusch said:

The act of administering medication, or thinking a child has received medication, may induce positive expectancies in parents and teachers about the effects of that medication, which may, in turn, influence how parents and teachers evaluate and behave toward children with ADHD. We speculate that the perception that a child is receiving ADHD medication may bring about a shift in attitude in a teacher or caregiver. They may have a more positive view of the child, which could create a better relationship. They may praise the child more, which may induce better behavior.[33]

The British article by John Naish concludes:

The more we believe in ADHD, the more we see it, the more we dose children with potentially dangerous drugs without monitoring them for dangerous responses. This latter concern is shared by Professor Peter Helms, a professor of child health at Aberdeen University, who . . . says that "The effects on people who have been on the drugs for years is a potential problem. Clinical trials give us only short-term answers, as the results last a year at most. We should introduce monitoring systems to check what is happening with patients."

Indeed, one important study in 2010 found that there are no benefits to giving children medication after they have been taking the drug for three years.

British GPs [general practitioners] agree that many are left on [ADD drugs] for more than three years, and often for as many as six years.

Furthermore, there is also disturbing evidence from studies on laboratory rats that giving [these types of] drugs to adolescents may cause them mental problems when they are adults. These may include memory damage and depression. In humans there have been no studies to explore this, because it is illegal to test drugs on children.

Instead, something else is happening: we're effectively witnessing an uncontrolled chemical trial that involves the mass medication of thousands of youngsters across Britain. What is even more tragic is that we are not even trying to monitor these children for earlier evidence of the serious problems in many cases.[34]

SODIUM NITRATE AND NITRITE

Sodium nitrate and nitrite are preservatives that are added to processed meat products such as bacon, corned beef, ham, hot dogs, sausage, and lunch meats for the purpose of preventing the growth of bacteria and to give the meat a deceptively healthy look. These compounds transform into cancer-causing agents, nitrosamines, in the stomach.

Nitrates and nitrites occur naturally in food and water but are also created chemically for fertilizers and preservatives. However, we get the most exposure to nitrates in food. One source said that the "nitrate intake from a typical U.S. diet provides an average of 75 to 100 mg per day of nitrate. Vegetables, particularly spinach, celery, beets, lettuce, and root vegetables, are responsible for most of the dietary intake. . . . The body also makes approximately 62 mg/day of nitrate in addition to what is ingested."[35]

The most risk from nitrates comes as a result of conversion to nitrite, with the highest danger coming from contaminated well water. Nitrate is converted to nitrite through the saliva in people, but infants convert nitrate to nitrite at double the rate of adults. The short-term effect is what nitrites do to the blood. They change the normal form of hemoglobin (which carries oxygen to the body) into something called methemoglobin that cannot carry oxygen.

If there is enough nitrate in drinking water, it can cause a temporary blood disorder in tiny babies called methemoglobinemia, "blue baby syndrome." This could cause brain damage or even death from suffocation because of lack of oxygen in babies up to six months of age. The New Hampshire Department of Environmental Services says that healthy adults do not develop this blood/oxygen disorder at nitrate levels in drinking water that puts infants at risk. However, adults exposed to this amount of nitrate can be affected with symptoms of dizziness, headaches, irritability, and blue tones around the eyes, mouth, hands, and feet, according to the health website iLunchBox.com. [36]

Of course there is the exposure to nitrates and nitrites when they are used to preserve meats and maintain a healthy color and flavor. Combining with amino acids in the stomach's acidic environment results in N-nitrosamines, known carcinogens. There is this helpful fact: vitamins C, D, and E inhibit the conversion of nitrites to nitrosamines in the stomach.[37] So, if you have to have bacon, squeeze yourself some orange juice to go along with it.

Eating a lot of meat products with nitrate preservatives, even with orange juice, is actually dangerous. The University of Southern California School of Medicine did a case-control study of children from birth to age 10 in Los Angeles County. With 232 cases and 232 controls, they tracked food items. Breakfast meats (bacon, sausage, ham); luncheon meats (salami, pastrami, lunch meat, corned beef, bologna); hot dogs; oranges and orange juice; and grapefruit and grapefruit juice. Also, they asked about consumption of apples and apple juice, regular and charbroiled meats, milk, coffee, and cola drinks. When risks were adjusted, the only significant find was that children eating more than 12 hot dogs per month have nine times the normal risk of developing childhood leukemia.[38]

Will eating a hot dog at a ball game kill you? Probably not. But eating a steady diet of nitrate-preserved meat might.

Sugars

Let's also look at refined sugars. The average American consumes 150 to 175 pounds of sugar per year. People are consuming half a cup of sugar a day, and most aren't even aware of it. Why? Because so much of it is in the food products they consume. The insidious nature of processed foods means sugar can virtually be found in all processed foods—unless they say sugar-free. If it says sugar-free, read the label carefully and look for the synthetic sweetener that's in it.

According to the World Health Organization (WHO), in November 2012, about 347 million people worldwide have diabetes.[39] The incidence of diabetes in the U.S. was 6.8 million in 1987, 18.5 million in 2000, 20.8 million in 2005, and 25.8 million in 2011.

The consumption of sugar and corresponding elevated insulin levels also causes weight gain, bloating, migraines, arthritis, fatigue, reduced immune function, creating gallstones, kidney stones, obesity, cancer, gum disease, cavities, and cardiovascular diseases, Alzheimer's, Lou Gehrig's, and dementia.

We know that many children today have been raised on sugar. It's even put in the formulas fed to them at birth by mothers who don't nurse. The infants consume significantly lower amounts of protein and have decreased amounts of B vitamins, iron, zinc, and vitamin E, all which are essential for brain, heart, and tissue development.

Bacteria overgrowth, candida, is a result from eating too many processed foods, sugars, and sugar replacements like aspartame and other cancer-causing sweeteners that are used for sugar replacements and in dietary foods that are recommended for diabetics.

Sugar comes in many forms, including dextrose, glucose, fructose, lactose, high fructose corn syrup, maple syrup, invert sugar, maltose, diastase, sorbitol, caramel, date sugar, dextrin, fruit juice, fruit juice concentrate, ethyl maltol, maltodextrin, sorghum syrup, and more.

HFCS. High fructose corn syrup is a sweetener made from genetically modified corn in a chemical process that uses two genetically modified enzymes. It is used in baked goods, breakfast cereals, candies, cookies, cakes, fruits, ice cream, jams, gelatins, salad dressings, soda pop, soups, and many other processed foods.

Will Allen of the Organic Consumers Union checked U.S. obesity maps on the CDC website. He writes that in 1985, 40 U.S. states had no obesity, 12 others had levels below 10 percent, and only 8 states had obesity in the 10 to 12 percent range. By 2011, only 11 states were at a 20-24 percent obesity range, 37 states had obesity above 25 percent, and 12 states had obesity above 30 percent—all in 26 years![40]

He further writes:

In a St. Louis University study on rats—fed the same diet that U.S. consumers eat—researchers reported that "we had a feeling we'd see evidence of fatty liver disease by the end of the study, but we were surprised to find how severe the damage was and how quickly it occurred. It took only four weeks for liver enzymes to increase and for glucose intolerance—the beginning of type II diabetes—to begin."[41] Scientists have concluded that this new sweetener—that humans had never ingested previously in human history—is a significant factor in our overweight/obesity/diabetic epidemic."[42]

Diabetes here we come.

MORE TOXINS

Here are more toxins that are found in our food supply.

Alginic Acid. This is also called algin or alginate, and it's used in the production of gel-like foods. The health food store has all kinds of things with this from hummus to cheese dips and vegetable dips. Alginic acid is also used to make antacids. But it is said to have a chalky taste and may cause you to have constipation, diarrhea, nausea, or vomiting.

BHA and BHT. These two toxins, BHA and BHT, were supposedly banned in the 70s or 80s in the U.S. Then manufacturers put them in the food packaging, which absorbs from the package into the food. How clever. They block the process of oil rancidity, which occurs when oil ages, is exposed to light, or has repeated exposure to air. These additives seem to affect sleep and appetite and have been associated with liver and kidney damage, baldness, behavior problems, cancer, fetal abnormalities, and growth retardation. Wow. Affect the sleep?

People with autism have disturbed sleep. Adults with PTSD have trouble with sleeping and anxiety. Any correlation?

What about the rations that the military feeds our soldiers? How many rations contain BHA and BHT to preserve them over months or years? These rations are also used by firefighters and as emergency rations. How many of them contain artificial dyes? They are all there. Many of the granolas sold in health food stores contain BHA or BHT as a preserving agent for granolas and granola bars. Potato chips and major food nutrients use them as well.

BVO. Bromated vegetable oil, BVO, has been brought into our food industry to hold or suspend citrus flavor in soft drinks. It is not allowed in Europe or Japan. Thanks to a petition from a Mississippi teenager in May 2014, both Coke and Pepsi announced they were taking it out of their products, including Mountain Dew, Fanta, and PowerAde.

The Dr. Pepper Snapple Group has not said if it will remove BVO from Squirt, Sun Drop, or Sunkist Peach Soda.

The New York Times said this about the BVO controversy: "Brominated vegetable oil contains bromine, the element found in brominated flame retardants, used in things like upholstered furniture and children's products. Research has found brominate flame retardants building up in the body and breast milk, and animal and some human studies have linked them to neurological impairment, reduced fertility, changes in thyroid hormones and puberty at an earlier age."[43]

Carmine and Cochineal Extract. This is a pigment extracted from dried eggs and bodies of the female *Dactylopius coccus,* a beetle-like insect that preys on cactus plants. The Maya and Inca peoples made a cloth dye of these insects. It is still used as a dye for clothing today and added to food for its dark crimson color. It is found in artificial crabmeat, fruit juices, frozen fruit snacks, candy, and yogurt. This chemical is comprised of about 90 percent insect body fragments. Although the government receives very few complaints, some organizations are asking for a mandatory warning to label cochineal-colored foods.

Chlorpyrifos. Dr. David Bellinger, professor of neurology at Harvard Medical School, calculated that in the U.S., children of mothers who had been exposed to organophosphates, the most common agricultural pesticide, lost a total of 16.9 million IQ points due to this exposure.[44] The organophosphate chlorpyrifos cost

Dow Chemical over $700,000 in fines for "concealing more than 200 reports of poisoning related to chlorpyrifos."[45] The "very highly toxic" chemical is still used in agriculture on both food and non-food crops, in plant nurseries and greenhouses, and on golf courses.

Dicyclomine and Linaclotide. Dicyclomine is a very specific drug for irritable bowel syndrome, which is basically a functional disorder of the gastrointestinal tract that wreaks a lot of havoc in the system, resulting in a lot of discomfort with pain, bloating, excess gas, and cramping.

What contributes to irritable bowel syndrome?
- The two most common causes are enzyme deficiency and poor dietary management, meaning not having good nutrition intake such as fiber, salads, vegetables, greens, and fruits—fresh, not canned, preserved, or cooked to death.
- Hypersensitivity to pain from a full bowel or gas comes from the inability to digest. That symptom is enzyme deficiency in itself.
- Movement, the flow through the colon, is too fast or too slow. Fiber helps to regulate that.
- Poor absorption of sugars and poor absorption of acids in the foods are present because of enzyme deficiency.
- Reproductive hormones or neurotransmitters may be off balance in people with irritable bowel syndrome, and this comes back again to nutritional deficiencies. Reproductive imbalance and hormone imbalance can be a mineral, protein, or fat imbalance. This all comes from eating processed foods.

Dicyclomine helps reduce the symptoms of stomach and intestinal cramping and works by relaxing the muscles in the stomach and intestine and by slowing the natural movements of the gut. It belongs to a class of drugs known as anticholinergics and antispasmodics. This medication should not be given to children younger than six months of age because of the risk of serious side effects. Symptoms such as dizziness, vomiting, diarrhea, abdominal pain, sweating, flatulence, abnormal distension, infections, infestations, viral gastroenteritis, and headaches are very common, just to name a few.[46]

One more drug that is very common for irritable bowel syndrome is linaclotide, which is indicated for irritable bowel syndrome with constipation. In adults, common side effects include diarrhea, abdominal pain, gas, and bloating.

So we see that the drugs they use to treat the condition that already manifests in diarrhea, constipation, gas, and bloating—the very drugs they give the patients for that condition—create the same side effects. If you have gas, you want something that will eliminate gas, not create more. If you've got abdominal pain, you want to eliminate it, not increase it.

All of these prescription drugs contribute to the destruction of the natural flora in the GI tract, which most likely was absent in the first place because of eating processed foods and sugars and not having proper nutrition.

Fluoride. In the United States there is a huge push to put fluoride in all the water. Proponents make the claim that it's good for your teeth, despite warnings of the dangers of fluoride. There is increased risk of bone cancer in boys, it affects endocrine function, and it suppresses thyroid function. In 2012 Harvard researcher Philippe Grandjean reported that after an exhaustive study of Chinese research in both high-natural and low-natural fluoride areas that "children in high-fluoride areas had significantly lower IQ scores than those who lived in low-fluoride areas."[47]

In the U.S. in 2010, 41 percent of adolescents ages 12 to 15 had dental fluorosis, permanent stains on their teeth, from ingesting too much fluoride, an increase of over 400 percent in 60 years. How could they not? Fluoride has been forced into our drinking water, and it's in toothpastes and mouth rinses. There are even prescription fluoride supplements. Filter your water and read product labels![48]

The renowned researcher from the Department of Environmental Health, Harvard School of Public Health, Philippe Grandjean, just published a real shocker! **His study officially classified fluoride as a *neurotoxin*** in the March 2014 journal of *The Lancet*. This journal is the world's oldest and most prestigious peer-reviewed medical journal. This scientist, who is affiliated with the University of Southern Denmark and the Harvard School of Public Health, has **identified fluoride as being in the same category as the neurotoxins arsenic, mercury, and lead![49]** [Emphasis added]

Fluoride is now classified as a neurotoxin and in the same category as arsenic, mercury, and lead!

Glyphosate. Glyphosate makes common herbicides work against weeds. It interferes with the biochemistry of bacteria, simple as that. When we understand the effects of glyphosate and the negative impact on the body, we find it is insidious and manifests slowly over time.

We can see all the ways glyphosate contributes to the chronic diseases that occur with increasing frequency, as use of this herbicide has increased steadily since its introduction into the herbicide/pesticide world. Glyphosate kills plants by interfering with a biochemical pathway involved with the synthesis of amino acids called shikimate pathway. These pathways are not found in humans, but they are found in plants, which is why glyphosate kills weeds.

The bad news is that this pathway is also found in bacteria. We realize that humans depend on bacteria in the gastrointestinal tract to synthesize the essential amino acids that are the building blocks of proteins, tissues, hormones, and the immune system throughout our body. Without bacteria we would cease to exist. By interfering with the biochemistry of bacteria in our GI tract, consumption of glyphosate depletes essential amino acids and sets us up for a host of chronic health problems. Glyphosate depletes the amino acids tyrosine, tryptophan, and phenylalanine. The loss of these amino acids can be a contributing factor in obesity, depression, autism, inflammatory bowel disease, Alzheimer's disease, and Parkinson's.

Another thing to consider is that the same level of glyphosate that kills good bacteria was found in a study[50] to allow several harmful pathogens like *Salmonella* to grow successfully. Feed GMO corn to chickens and get more growth of *Salmonella?* And that's not all the bad news. A study done in cattle also found glyphosate killed the good bacteria, and the residues on cattle feed may predispose cattle to botulism infection.[51]

Companies should consider non-toxic weed killers that are made from essential oils! We do not have to poison the earth and ourselves with glyphosate.[52]

Heterocyclic Amines. Cooking meats at high temperatures creates the carcinogens heterocyclic amines. The National Cancer Institute at the National Institutes of Health reports that 17 different heterocyclic amines that result from cooking muscle meats are believed to have human cancer risk.[53] Enough said.

Hexane. Hexane is a byproduct of gasoline manufacturing. It is a neurotoxin and an air pollutant. It is not common knowledge but manufacturers soak soybeans in hexane to extract the oil (used to make soy protein). The Cornucopia Institute reports that a certain health bar is made with organic oats and soybeans and is legally allowed to be called "organic" because 70 percent of the soy IS organic. But the remaining 30 percent can be hexane extracted. The Cornucopia Institute sent a sample of hexane-extracted soy meal (used in those popular "health" bars) to an independent analytical laboratory that is registered with the FDA and the USDA. The soy meal contained 21 ppm (parts per million) of hexane.[54]

That may not sound like much, but in two foods that are required to be tested for hexane (soy products are NOT required), fish protein isolate can't have more than 5 ppm; and hop extract and spice resins can't have more than 25 ppm. Is 21 ppm something to worry about in soy meal? Soy meal is used for protein in infant formulas, veggie burgers, and energy bars. What do you think?

Hydrolyzed Vegetable Protein. HVT (also Textured Vegetable Protein—TVP) is the result of breaking down vegetables (the most common is soy) into their component amino acids. HVT allows food processors to achieve stronger flavors from fewer ingredients. It is one of many "flavoring" agents used in a sneaky way to get MSG into a food without having it on the label! Most often HVP is from GM soy and is found in canned soups, chili, frozen dinners, and beef- and chicken-flavored products.

Natural Health writer Mike Adams wrote: "HVP, TVP and yeast extract are very common ingredients in the natural/vegetarian food industry. Most of the popular veggie burgers, for example, contain HVP, TVP or yeast extract. And that makes them a suspected source of **hidden MSG**."[55]

Interesterified Fat. This fat was developed in response to demand for trans-fat alternatives, because trans fats increase your cholesterol and were basically banned. This semi fat is created by chemically blending fully hydrogenated and non-hydrogenated oils found in pastries, margarine, frozen dinners and canned soups. Some people say, "But it makes it easier to prepare supper." Easier, but surely a health problem. The early evidence doesn't look promising. A study by Malaysian researchers showed a four-week diet of 12 percent of interesterified fats increased the ratio of LDL and HDL cholesterol—not a good thing. The study also showed an increase in blood glucose levels and a decrease in insulin response. Watch out for diabetes.

Mono- and Di-Glycerides. Mono- and di-glycerides are fats added to foods to bind liquids with fats. They occur naturally in foods and constitute about 1 percent of normal fats. They are found in everything from breads, breakfast pastries, baked goods, mashed potatoes, peanut butter, ice cream, and margarine. These are very typical and found in most of your vegetarian/vegan products, particularly in whole-grain and multi-grain breads. These are also a derivative of animal fat, often simply labeled "vegetable monodiglycerides." So beware. "Vegetable" monodiglycerides can come from animal fat.

Olestra. Some potato chips still have this fat substitute, but it is not very popular because of "leakage." From 1996 until 2003, the FDA required this warning: "This Product Contains Olestra. Olestra may cause abdominal cramping and loose stools [diarrhea]. Olestra inhibits the absorption of some vitamins and other nutrients. Vitamins A, D, E, and K have been added." Afraid that the warning was scaring away customers, a petition from the manufacturer got the warning removed.

Olestra passes through the body undigested because its molecules are so large. In the process, the fat soluble A, D, E, K, and others attach to the substance, thinking it is a fat, and are inadvertently flushed out of the body, causing vitamin deficiencies.

It can cause diarrhea and anal leakage, which can be part of irritable bowel syndrome and may contribute to leaky gut syndrome. It can sometimes still be found on grocery shelves.

PCBs. Polychlorinated biphenyls (PCBs) are continually being found in the environment, especially in rivers, even though they were banned in the U.S. in 1976. However, an estimated 250 million pounds of these oily fluids are still legally in service today in "totally enclosed uses," largely as transformers and capacitors. The Environmental Protection Agency has identified many sites where the chemicals have been illegally dumped or accidentally spilled. It is an environmental imperative that they all be removed. PCBs cause many adverse health effects in humans and are known to impact the nervous, reproductive, endocrine, and immune systems of fish and birds. Just imagine what they do to us.

Propyl Lactate. Propyl lactate is a preservative that is used to prevent fats and oils from spoiling. It is often combined with BHT and BHA. The side effects that have been found in animal studies show that propyl lactate has been linked to cancer. Possible reactions in humans include asthma attacks, allergic reactions, liver and kidney damage, and gastric irritation.

VACCINES

Vaccine promoters love to show you graphs of disease rates in the UK, the United States, and Australia that show conclusively that vaccines are responsible for saving millions of lives. What they don't show you is that the disease rates were *already* in a steep decline because of improved hygiene. An editorial in the *Journal of Pediatrics* states that proper sanitation was largely responsible for the early large declines in infectious diseases: ". . . the largest historical decrease in morbidity and mortality caused by infectious disease was experienced not with the modern antibiotic and vaccine era, but after the introduction of clean water and effective sewer systems."[56]

So the promoters are not exactly being truthful. What else do they twist to their purposes?

Autism and Vaccines

Dr. Andrew Wakefield was a surgeon and gastroenterology researcher at the Royal Free Hospital in London when in 1998, he announced at a press conference the results of his study. It gave him strong concerns about the safety of the measles, mumps, and rubella vaccine (MMR) and its relationship to the onset of autism. So what was the outcome of this man just trying to bring an awareness that in his work as a physician he saw things that caused him alarm and concern?

They pulled this man's license and branded him as a quack. *The Lancet*, which published the original Wakefield study, retracted it. Do a search and you will read inflammatory and derogatory statements like this one from Wikipedia: "Andrew Wakefield has become one of the most reviled doctors of his generation, blamed directly and indirectly, depending on the accuser, for irresponsibly starting a panic with triggering repercussions, vaccination rates so low that childhood diseases, once all but eradicated—whooping cough and measles among them—have re-emerged, endangering young lives."[57]

The popular press sure won't tell you the truth of how Wakefield was slandered and the lies that have been told about his research.

In 2011, the *British Medical Journal* quoted research microbiologist David Lewis, who explained that he reviewed grading sheets of two of Dr. Wakefield's 1998 co-authors, pathologists Amar Dhillon and Andrew Anthony, which led him to the conclusion that there was **no fraud** committed by Dr. Wakefield.

In a press release, Lewis stated: "The grading sheets and other evidence in Wakefield's files clearly show that it is unreasonable to conclude, based on a comparison of the histological records, that Andrew Wakefield 'faked' a link between MMR vaccine and autism."[58]

Have you read about this on the Internet? In other news articles? As we all know and have watched for years, if there's a threat to somebody's pocketbook, the first thing they usually do is to attack the messenger.

In a 2006 British newspaper article, Dr. Wakefield said, "The Department of Health and some of the media wanted to dismiss our research as insignificant. The excuse was that no one else had the same findings as us. What they didn't say is that no one else looked."[59]

The same British newspaper article that quoted Dr. Wakefield told about a Wake Forest University School of Medicine research team that set out to examine 275 children with regressive autism; and of the 82 they had tested at that time, 70 proved positive for the measles virus in their gastrointestinal tract. The study leader, Dr. Stephen Walker, told the newspaper, "What it means is that the study done earlier by Dr. Wakefield and published in 1998 is correct."[60]

Well, 28 other studies looked at the gastrointestinal problems of autistic children and confirmed Dr. Wakefield's study.

Of the 28 studies that confirm what Dr. Wakefield found in autistic children, I will quote just two. From the journal *Pediatric Neurology*.

> The level of measles antibody, but not mumps or rubella antibodies, was significantly higher in autistic children as compared to normal children. . . . autistic children have a hyper-immune response to measles virus, which in the absence of a wild-type measles infection might be a sign of an abnormal immune reaction to the vaccine strain or virus reactivation.[61]

The University of Maryland School of Medicine in Baltimore did a study on autistic children's gastrointestinal abnormalities. The study authors were not afraid to mention the work of Dr. Wakefield: "The report of Wakefield, et al represents the first effort to evaluate the gastrointestinal tract in children with autism." Further in the study, the authors again quoted Wakefield and his co-authors: "They performed colonoscopy with histological examinations in 12 children and reported that all had intestinal abnormalities. . . ."[62]

The 28 studies suggest that there certainly may be a link between the MMR vaccine, bowel disease, and autism.[63]

So, the *real* guinea pigs, the *real* test subjects, are humans. Yet when the humans cry out and say vaccines are creating autism, then the government goes into full-fledged battle to prove that vaccines are safe and do not cause autism.

The Centers for Disease Control just announced that now 1 in every 68 children is autistic, a nearly 30 percent climb in rates.[64] Since the turn of the century, autism rates have more than doubled. With all the toxins our children are exposed to, are we surprised?

Additional Worries About Vaccines

An interesting thing happened in July 2013. The Centers for Disease Control was a little too honest in admitting that up to 98 million Americans received polio vaccine contaminated with the cancer-linked monkey virus SV40 (Simian Virus 40). Sayer Ji, who founded GreenMediaInfo.com, said that sometime after July 11, 2013, the page disappeared.[65] Did too many people start to complain? Did you know about this?

Polio vaccine was produced in rhesus monkey kidney cells. Lucky for monkeys, the virus is dormant in them; not so in humans. Here is the gist of the now-missing CDC text:

- SV40 is a virus found in some species of monkey.
- SV40 was discovered in 1960. Soon afterward, the virus was found in polio vaccine.
- More than 98 million Americans received one or more doses of polio vaccine from 1955 to 1963 when a proportion of vaccine was contaminated with SV40; it has been estimated that 10-30 million Americans could have received an SV40 contaminated dose of vaccine.
- SV40 virus has been found in certain types of cancer in humans, but it has not been determined that SV40 causes these cancers.
- The majority of scientific evidence suggests that SV40-contaminated vaccine did not cause cancer; however, some research results are conflicting and more studies are needed.
- Polio vaccines today do not contain SV40. All of the current evidence indicates that polio vaccines have been free of SV40 since 1963.

Sayer Ji says that the virus was only in the injected polio vaccine and that vaccines produced by the former Soviet Union until 1980 exposed hundreds of millions more people in the USSR, China, Japan, and several African countries to the virus.

Ji says that SV40 is really just the tip of the iceberg being "only one of a wide range of so-called 'adventitious' viruses that continue to contaminate vaccine seed stock and substrate (cells used to grow vaccine), which include **endogenous retroviruses** such as mouse mammary tumor virus, and many which have yet to be identified. SV40 was after all **the 40th** simian virus identified, and this was 50 years ago. We can only imagine how many hidden disease vectors exist and have been identified by vaccinologists and virologists over the intervening years but which never made it to the light of day."[66] [Emphasis in the original]

The CDC is not being entirely truthful by saying it hasn't been determined that SV40 causes the cancers it is found in. Sayer Ji says SV40 suppresses a protein in humans that protects against the initiation of cancer.

Do you think this is the only problem in vaccines? Of course not. There is more data you need to learn about.

Vaccine Fillers

In addition to viral bacterial RNA or DNA that is part of the vaccines, here are the fillers: aluminum hydroxide, aluminum phosphate, ammonium sulfate, amphotericin B; animal tissues: pig blood, horse blood, rabbit brain, dog kidney, monkey kidney, chick embryo, chicken egg, duck egg, calf (bovine) serum, betapropiolactone, fetal bovine serum, formaldehyde, formalin, gelatin, glycerol, human diploid cells (originating from human aborted fetal tissue), hydrolyzed gelatin, monosodium glutamate (MSG), neomycin, neomycin sulfate, phenol red indicator, phenoxyethanol (antifreeze), potassium diphosphate, potassium monophosphate, polymyxin B, polysorbate 20, polysorbate 80, porcine (pig) pancreatic hydrolysate of casein, residual MRC5 proteins, sorbitol, sucrose, **thimerosal (mercury),** tri(n)butylphosphate, VERO cells, a continuous line of monkey kidney cells, washed sheep red blood cells.[67] [Emphasis in original]

Are Vaccinations the Solution?

How often do we hear that this or that outbreak would not have happened if all kids were vaccinated? Yet in the *Journal of the American Medical Association* (November, 1990), it stated: "Although more than 95% of school-age children in the United States are vaccinated against measles, large measles outbreaks continue to occur in schools, and in most cases in this setting occur among **previously vaccinated children**."[68] [Emphasis added]

The medical solution? Just keep revaccinating! Our solution? If vaccines don't work, let's get rid of them!

Do your homework before you accept any vaccines for yourself or your family. Do you know that flu vaccines still contain the mercury-based preservative thimerosal? Thimerosal is 50 percent mercury by weight, and that's from the FDA. A University of Calgary video shows how mercury kills brain cells. You can see it now on YouTube at http://www.youtube.com/watch?v-tC9BPAF0dEA. Watch this and think about your brain cells before you accept a flu shot.[69]

FROGS IN A POT

Are we like frogs in a pot of cold water where someone turns on the stove and slowly cooks us? Do we believe that all is well and that if something was wrong, our governments would tell us? Do we live with our head in the sand and wonder why we don't feel well and why all diseases are on the increase? Unfortunately, the vast majority of people today do not read, know about, or believe what's going on with the world's food supply.

People gladly consume aspartame, fluoride, and BPA, (a hormone-disrupting chemical used in plastic bottles and in the lining of canned foods). Pesticides, high fructose corn syrup, pharmaceutical drugs, and toxic vaccines with disastrous side effects they don't even question. Then when their child displays a change in behavior, they go to the doctor crying, "What happened? It didn't happen 'til after my child was vaccinated."

Often, the doctor then replies, "Oh, the vaccine would have had nothing to do with it; it's strictly a coincidence."

But the fact is and remains that our children are getting sicker and sicker younger and younger every year. The mental disorder of our children is at an epidemic level throughout the world.

I travel the world and see people in many countries. For example, children in the jungles of the Amazon who are not exposed to the toxic foods and chemicals are healthy, bright, and vibrant. Their eyes are dancing. They're not dull and listless, and they haven't been shot full of vaccines, yet they haven't been sick either. They live off the land.

I have been in dozens of villages that I had to get to in a canoe through tributaries off the Amazon in Peru and Ecuador. These people get to the outside world sometimes once every two or three years at best, and it's too difficult to bring processed food back. They live off the land, on what they can gather, on food from their gardens, and their animals that they raise. In so many villages that I stopped in, the villagers had chickens, goats, pigs, and/or a cow. They raised their own meat and had gardens. Every single village had gardens. These people were healthy, they looked healthy, their energy was vibrant, their hair was beautiful, and they had good teeth.

As I visited the villages in the interior of Somalia and ate with some families, they didn't serve me bread, coffee, or soda pop. They served me goat liver and onions. They raised the goat and the onions came from a vegetable garden. I drank clabbered buttermilk from their goats. It was delicious to me because I grew up on it. These people weren't dying of cancer, and the children in those villages didn't have autism; they also weren't vaccinated.

One report states that the United States is now in 35th place in the world in overall life expectancy. That's probably being very conservative.[70] What's happened to our food chain in the last hundred years? Our foods and drinks are contaminated with chemicals and toxins. Curiously, government food authorities shamelessly promote these chemicals and continue to endorse them being put in our food chain and in our animal feed as well.

We must read labels and avoid foods with additives and chemicals. We must stand up and protect our families. We must let our stores know that we want to buy foods without additives and chemicals. I go into health food stores and can see as much toxic food as good food. I kind of chuckle, as I've said to store managers, "I thought this was a health food place, and yet you're selling as much sugar as the grocery stores."

Of course people want to believe that our government is concerned about our well-being, while the food producers and manufacturers lead us to believe that these food additives are to improve the nutritional value of our foods by "enriching" and "enhancing" them, yet the very ingredients in them are stripping the nutrients out of our bodies and setting us up to be victims of irritable bowel syndrome, fibromyalgia, arthritis, diabetes, cancer, or heart disease.

IT'S UP TO YOU

It's tempting to stick our head in the sand and overlook these troublesome issues. Toxicity studies on laboratory animals are typically short term, and they don't weigh all the variables that are taken into consideration like dosages and isolations and whether they are feeding the rats the same diet that humans are eating. Unfortunately, the human diet is so much worse!

What would tests show if mice or rats lived on the diets children do for the first 18 years of their life? What if they lived on hamburger helper, sugar-coated cereals, macaroni and cheese, and all the foods that are filled with chemical flavorings, extenders, binders, and hybrid gluten that are terrorizing their intestinal tract? Add to this the emotional stress that triggers more inflammation. It's like the body is a time bomb just ticking away with all the chemicals.

The solution is simple: Eat as natural as possible, avoid additives, and be a label reader.

ENDNOTES

1   http://www.pewhealth.org/projects/food-additives-project-85899367220.
2   Lau K, et al. Synergistic interactions between commonly used food additives in a developmental neurotoxicity test. *Toxicol Sci.* 2006 Mar;90(1):178-87.
3   Hull JS. *Sweet Poison, How the World's Most Popular Artificial Sweetener Is Killing Us—My Story—.* New Horizon Press, 1999.
4   http://www.ewg.org/research/nearly-500-ways-make-yoga-mat-sandwich.
5   http://preventdisease.com/news/13/091013_This-Ingredient-Is-Found-In-Most-Cereals-Bread-and-Foamed-Plastics-and-Rubber-Too.shtml.
6   http://www.huffingtonpost.com/2014/02/07/subway-chemical-azodicarbonamide-bread_n_4746304.html.
7   http://www.ext.colostate.edu/pubs/foodnut/09371.pdf.
8   Grant J. List of Foods Containing GMOs. LIVESTRONG.COM. Dec. 17, 2013. http://www.livestrong.com/article/314824-list-of-foods-containing-gmos/.
9   http://foodmatters.tv/articles-1/gm-corn-linked-to-cancer-tumors.
10 Séralini GE, et al. Long term toxicity of a Roundup herbicide and a Roundup-tolerant genetically modified maize. *Food Chem Toxicol.* 2012 Nov;50(11):4221-31.
11 Ibid.
12 http://www.truthinlabeling.org/IVhistoryOfUse.html.
13 http://www.truthinlabeling.org/manufac.html.
14 http://www.dorway.com/blayenn.html.
15 Coyle JT, et al. Excitatory amino acid neurotoxins: selectivity, specificity, and mechanisms of action. Based on an NRP one-day conference held June 30, 1980. *Neurosci Res Program Bull.* 1081;19(4):1-427.
16 Olney JW. Brain lesions, obesity, and other disturbances in mice treated with monosodium glutamate. *Science.* 1969 May 9;164(38890):719-21.
17 http://www.dorway.com/blayenn.html.
18 Ibid.
19 http://jn.nutrition.org/content/125/11/2891S.full.pdf.

20 http://articles.mercola.com/sites/articles/archive/2009/04/21/msg-is-this-silent-killer-lurking-in-your-kitchen-cabinets.aspx.

21 http://www.epa.gov/pesticides/food/risks.htm.

22 Weldon RH, Barr DB, Trujillo C, Bradman A, Holland N, Eskenazi B. A Pilot Study of Pesticides and PCBs in the Breast Milk of Women Residing in Urban and Agricultural Communities of California. *J Environ Monit.* 2011 Nov;13(11):3136-44.

23 Lim JS, et al. Inverse associations between long-term weight change and serum concentrations of persistent organic pollitants. *Int J Obes* (London). 2011 May;35(5):744-7.

24 http://epa.gov/ncer/science/endocrine/pdf/development/r826131_veeramachaneni_0415.pdf.

25 Sengupta P, Bannerjee R. Environmental toxins: Alarming impacts of pesticides on male fertility. *Hum Exp. Toxicol.* 2013 Dec 17. ACOG Committee Opinion No 575. Exposure to toxic environmental agents. *Fertil Steril.* 2013 Oct;100(4):931-4.

26 http://www.iol.co.za/lifestyle/family/kids/are-our-kids-ritalin-guinea-pigs-1.1292850#.U3DsvDhOWUk.

27 Ibid.

28 Ibid.

29 Ibid.

30 Thurstone C, et al. Randomized, controlled trial of atomoxetine for attention-deficit/hyperactivity disorder in adolescents with substance use disorder. *J Am Acad Child Adolesc Psychiatry.* 2010 Jun;49(6):573-82.

31 http://www.strattera.com/safety-information-adult-adhd-treatment.aspx.

32 Ibid.

33 Waschbusch DA, et al. Are there placebo effects in the medication treatment of children with attention-deficit hyperactivity disorder? *J Dev Behav Pediatr.* 2009 Apr;30(2):158-68. http://www.buffalo.edu/news/releases/2009/06/10217.html.

34 http://www.iol.co.za/lifestyle/family/kids/are-our-kids-ritalin-guinea-pigs-1.1292850#.U3DsvDhOWUk.

35 New Hampshire Department of Environmental Services, Environmental Fact Sheet, ARD-EHP-16.

36 Ibid.

37 Mirvish SS. Experimental evidence for inhibition of N-nitroso compound formation as a factor in the negative correlation between vitamin C consumption and the incidence of certain cancers. *Cancer Res.* 1994 Apr 1;54(7 Suppl):1948s-1951s.

38 Peters JM, et al. Processed meats and risks of childhood leukemia (California, USA). *Cancer Causes Control.* 1994 Mar;5(2):195-202.

39 http://www.healthcommunities.com/understanding-diabetes/diabetes-incidence-prevalence.shtml.

40 http://www.organicconsumers.org/articles/article_26209.cfm.

41 Ibid.

42 http://observationpost42.com/_Supersize_Me__Mice_Researc...pdf.

43 http://www.nytimes.com/2012/12/13/business/another-look-at-a-drink-ingredient-brominated-vegetable-oil.html?adxnnl=1&pagewanted=all&adxnnlx=1356247075-ofsnEpX9vqp4LrvhH2hbxg&_r=0.

44 Belliner DC. A strategy for comparing the contributions of environmental chemicals and other risk factors to neurodevelopment of children. *Environ Health Perspect.* 2012 Apr;120(4):501-7.

45 Hamblin J. The Toxins That Threaten Our Brains. *Atlantic Monthly,* March 2014. http://www.theatlantic.com/features/archive/2014/03/the-toxins-that-threaten-our-brains/284466/.

46 http://www.nlm.nih.gov/medlineplus/druginfo/meds/a684007.html.

47 Choi AL, Grandjean P, et al. Developmental fluoride neurotoxicity: a systematic review and meta-analysis. *Environ Health Perspect.* 2012 Oct;120(10):1362-8.

48 http://fluoridealert.org/issues/fluorosis/.

49 Grandjean P, Landrigan PJ. Neurobehavioural effects of developmental toxicity. *Lancet Neurol.* 2014 Mar;13(3):330-8.

50 Shehata AA, et al. The Effect of glyphosate on potential pathogens and beneficial members of poultry microbiota in vitro. *Curr Microbiol.* 2013 Apr;66(4):350-8.

51 Krüger M, et al. Glyphosate suppresses the antagonistic effect of Enterococcus spp. on *Clostridum botulinum. Anaerobe.* 2013 Apr;20:74-8.

52 http://www.dgaryyoung.com/blog/2013/developing-organic-weed-and-pest-control/.

53 http://www.cancer.gov/cancertopics/factsheet/Risk/cooked-meats.

54 http://www.cornucopia.org/soysurvey/OrganicSoyReport/behindthebean_color_final.pdf.

55 http://www.naturalnews.com/028323_Hydrolyzed_Vegetable_Protein_HVP.html.

56 Zinc, diarrhea, and pneumonia (editorial). *J Pediatr.* 1999 Dec;135(6):663.

57 http://en.wikipedia.org/wiki/Andrew Wakefield.

58 http://articles.mercola.com/sites/articles/archive/2012/01/24/new-evidence-refutes-fraud-findings-in-dr-wakefield-case.aspx.

59 http://www.dailymail.co.uk/news/article-388051/Scientists-fear-MMR-link-autism.html.

60 Ibid.

61 Singh VK, Jensen RL. Elevated Levels of Measles Antibodies in Children with Autism. *Pediatr Neurol.* 2003 Apr;28(4):292-4.

62 Horvath K, et al. Gastrointestinal abnormalities in children with autistic disorder. *J Pediatr.* 1999 Nov;135(5):559-63.

63 http://articles.mercola.com/sites/articles/archive/2010/04/10/wakefield-interview.aspx.

64 http://www.cdc.gov/ncbddd/autism/facts.html.

65 http://www.greenmedinfo.com/blog/cdc-disappears%E2%80%99-page-linking-polio-vaccines-cancer-causing-viruses1.

66 Ibid.

67 http://articles.mercola.com/sites/articles/archive/2001/03/07/vaccine-ingredients.aspx.

68 Mast EE, et al. Risk factors for measles in a previously vaccinated population and cost-effectiveness of revaccination strategies. *JAMA.* 1990 Nov 21;264(19):2529-33.

69 http://www.youtube.com/watch?v=tC9BPAF0dEA.

70 http://en.wikipedia.org/wiki/List_of_countries_by_life_expectancy.

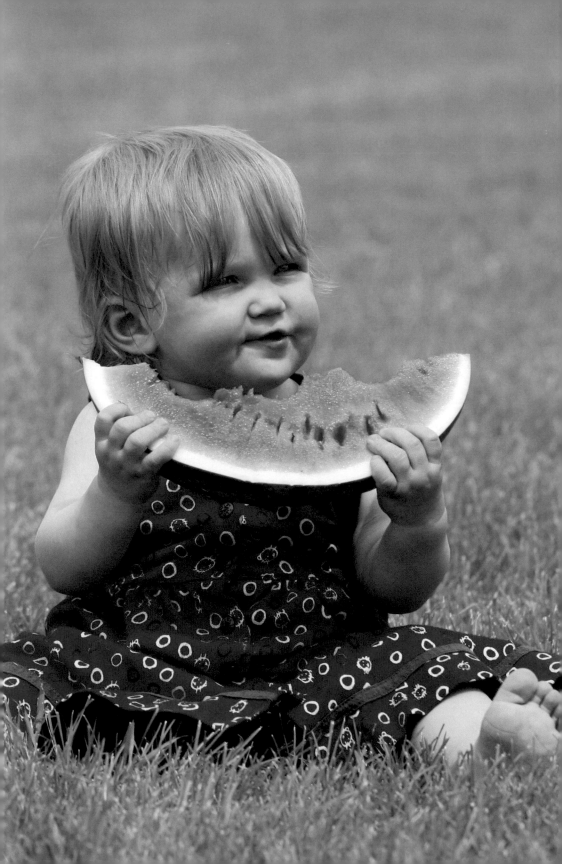

CHAPTER 8

The Road to Recovery and a Healthy Life

Looking for the answers to our modern-day diseases and how those answers link back to the ancient world of wheat has been a fascinating time of research and discovery. I have learned so much that has changed the way we eat in our home. Even our boys have become label readers and are quite careful about what they want to buy at the health food store.

Beware: Not all foods sold in the health food stores are healthful foods to eat. Many contain chemicals and other non-nutritious ingredients. Marketing is very clever these days, so we must be very selective in our shopping.

EINKORN, THE SUPER FOOD — A FULL CIRCLE

My study of wheat has brought me full circle from the wheat that we grew on our family's ranch more than 60 years ago to my discovery and cultivation of einkorn on my farms today. I appreciate more and more my farming background and my knowledge of growing and harvesting.

We were excited when the first shipment of einkorn flour came from our farm in France over a year ago and have had a lot of fun creating einkorn recipes. Trial and error serves us well for discovering what works and what doesn't, and I have learned a lot about different grains and flours being used today.

I believe that many people are going to really enjoy eating whole-grain einkorn bread and other einkorn products because of their delightful taste and wonderful nutrition. I'm sure many new recipes will be created, and many fun stories about baking with einkorn will be shared.

Whole-grain einkorn, still in its original structure, easily takes the lead in nutrition with twice the vitamin A content of modern wheat, three to four times more beta-carotene, four to five times more riboflavin, and three to four times more lutein. These nutrients, known to boost immunity, will help keep the body strong and are heart-healthy and supportive of eye health.

This ancient wheat is probably the most nutritious grain that has ever been grown. Even today, no other grain shows the nutritional value, the balance of proteins, and a glycemic index of 65, compared to white wheat flour with an index of 85.[1] "One tablespoon of wheat flour will spike blood sugar two times faster and higher than one tablespoon of white sugar."[2]

I have been interested to see that in the last four years, since 2010 when I first started talking about and researching einkorn, sites about it are popping up all over the Internet claiming to be growing einkorn in Montana, Washington, Idaho, and a big producer in Italy.

The challenge with knowing what is actually being grown in Italy is that farmers grow emmer, spelt, and einkorn and often call them all "farro"—emmer (*Triticum dicoccum*) is called "farro medio" or "true farro"; spelt (*Triticum spelta*) is called "farro grande" and is considered to be a "fake farro"; and einkorn (*Triticum monococcum*) is called "farro piccolo," "faricella," or "little farro" and is also considered to be a "fake farro." This has caused widespread confusion, so knowing whether the grain you are buying from Italy is actually einkorn is a challenge.

I ordered seed from two different growers in Washington who claimed to be growing einkorn, and it was spelt. I ordered seed from another company that also claimed to be growing einkorn, and it was kamut.

How does the public know what it is buying? How long will farmers continue to grow and harvest the hybrid wheat? How long will the rise of disease, allergies, gluten intolerance, celiac disease, and so many others continue to increase? When you have a possible answer, you need to speak out. You need to warn people. Our world is highly inundated with food void of nutrition and filled with chemicals. When we see children—even babies—drinking soda pop and eating candy and ice-cream, we have to ask ourselves, "What will be the outcome of this diet? What suffering will these children experience when they are teenagers and adults?

We have to wonder that if man can be so innovative as to travel to the moon or invent a cell phone where you can talk to somebody or send a message in a matter of seconds around the world, why can't we invent mechanized equipment that would process our grains the old way, allowing them to mature, germinate, and activate the enzymes that will render a sustainable food for the human body in a harmonic and healthful way?

Einkorn flour has a little bit of a tannish color and actually has a sweeter taste than regular wheat flour. The polysaccharide content of wheat flour will spike the glucose in the human body 3.5 times higher than white sugar, but the polysaccharide content of einkorn flour is much lower. The einkorn gluten content is so much lower that it is harder to make bread with it because it doesn't rise very well. You have to experiment with the yeast a little bit and with a sweetener like yacon or agave to get it to culture before mixing it into your dough.

Baked bread, pastries, pancakes, muffins, rolls, etc., made with einkorn are light and fluffy and have a wonderful taste. You don't get a bloated or stuffed feeling or feel uncomfortable. In fact, if you eat too fast, you might overeat because you don't get a sense of being too full. Einkorn is not acidic but it is nutritious and healing to the body.

You can experiment with einkorn flour by mixing it with a small amount of different flours such as brown rice, amaranth, sorghum, legumes, and/or graham flour from India that make it a good protein and highly nutritious. I have even mixed a little cacao powder into the flour to make chocolate pancakes, and that was a huge hit with the children.

If you find einkorn flour in the health food store, be sure to read the label carefully. In order to lengthen the shelf life, manufacturers will often remove most of the germ and bran, which contain most of the nutrition. Be sure to look for "whole-grain" einkorn flour.

Those who have gluten sensitivities or celiac disease should eat einkorn with caution. It is always best to try a little the first time or two just to see how your body reacts.

Take enzymes an hour before eating and a good probiotic at night before going to bed to build up the intestinal flora. Within time, the perforated mucosa of the gut can be repaired to where any individual should be able to go forward within a year or two and live a normal life.

A FEW SUGGESTIONS
Consider what you can change in your diet so that you can live a healthy life:

1. Think about what you are eating that may be causing inflammation and damaging your intestinal lining. These foods may include hybridized and GMO grains, especially hybrid wheat and corn; foods and beverages containing caffeine; alcohol; prepackaged and frozen meals; canned foods; and processed foods made with chemicals, fillers, and other hidden ingredients.

2. Stay away from foods that commonly cause allergies, including hybridized grains like wheat, corn, rye, barley, spelt, kamut, and others, etc.; milk products; soy; and refined sugars. The grains are fine if they are not hybridized GMO grains. Often the label will say, "Non-GMO" or "100% natural, non-GMO and/or gluten free." If you don't have that information on the label, then ask about the product before you buy it.

3. Read the labels carefully on all foods that say they are "gluten-free." These foods are often full of sugar, preservatives, food coloring, and many undesirable ingredients, perhaps even more undesirable than the gluten.

4. Eliminate foods made with sugar, artificial sweeteners, and "natural" flavorings. Beware of any ingredient that says "natural" because even chemicals can be natural. The word "natural" is often a cover up for many undesirable ingredients in the food and cosmetic industries. Natural flavorings may contain more chemicals than the artificial flavorings, food colorings, and preservatives. Again, be aware and try to avoid all unnatural and synthetic substances.

5. Do not eat non-organic foods that do not have a hard skin or shell and are porous like berries, apples, pears, tomatoes, beans, peas, carrots, broccoli, spinach, potatoes, onions, asparagus, etc. If they are not organic, they most likely have been sprayed or have some kind of chemical put on them; and those chemicals are easily absorbed into the food. Thick-rind produce like watermelon, squash, grapefruit, bananas, etc., might be edible; but if you have organic as a choice, don't choose non-organic.

6. Avoid foods, cosmetics, skin-care products, household cleaning products, etc., that contain chemicals.

7. Be a label reader. If there is something you don't understand, research it and find out what it means. Find out what you would be putting into your body.

8. If you are suffering with candida overgrowth, fungus, and parasites, look for non-chemical solutions and stop taking the non-steroidal, anti-inflammatory drugs (NSAIDs).

9. Increase the fiber in your diet by eating organic fruits such as apples, pears, and berries; vegetables such as broccoli and artichokes; nuts such as almonds; non-hybrid whole grains such as einkorn; and legumes.

10. Use sea salt instead of processed salt.

11. Take enzymes and high quality pre- and probiotics

12. Drink filtered or purified water, never chlorinated and/or fluoridated water. Many restaurants will tell you their water is filtered when it isn't. Some will tell you the chlorine is to prevent harmful bacteria. The safest is to ask for bottled water or mineral water. But do not drink water that is brought to your table in a pitcher unless you can verify that it goes through a filtering process first. Drinking water is extremely important because it helps flush toxins and increases enzyme saturation throughout the body tissues, as well as keeping you hydrated; but don't drink water that is going to put more toxins into your body.

13. Eat the best food you can. The better you eat, the better you will feel. Eat organic food, even though it may not be 100 percent organic. Although a farmer may be growing an organic crop, the farmer next to him may be growing a crop that is laden with toxic sprays that can travel through the air, contaminating the crops around his farm. There is no guarantee that organic food is truly organic, but it is definitely a better choice. Your best source is to plant and grow your own organic garden.

14. The U.S. federal regulations do not require full disclosure on product labels. The only way to avoid dangerous food additives is to eat whole, organic foods as much as possible and processed foods as little as possible.

15. Do your research on vaccinations. When searching on the Internet, type in "the dangers of vaccinations." If you just type in "vaccinations," what comes up may not show you that there is any danger. But danger there is and don't doubt it for a moment.

     When Mary birthed Jacob in the birthing center of our local hospital, the nurse came in with her cart to give him the standard vaccinations. I was ready to do battle when I told her he was not going to be vaccinated. Her face had a look of relief on it as she said, "Oh, thank you, Mr. Young." I was so surprised and asked her what she meant by that. She said that they see so many awful things happen with vaccinations, and she hated giving them to the babies. I asked her why she doesn't warn the parents, and she said that by law, she could **not** say anything. Does that tell a story? Beware and know the facts.

IT'S UP TO US

It is very easy to stick our head in the sand and pretend everything is going great. "It won't happen to me" is a typical attitude before the storm hits. Pollution and contamination are everywhere, and the degeneration of our society is staring us in the face.

Toxicity studies on laboratory animals are typically short term, often only a few months at best; and they don't weigh all the variables that are taken into consideration like dosages and isolations and whether they are feeding the rats the same diet that humans are eating. Unfortunately, the human diet is much worse!

What would tests show if mice or rats lived on the diets of our children for the first 18 years of their lives with packaged and frozen meals, sugar-coated cereals, macaroni and cheese, white bread, sugar, processed salt, pasteurized milk, "natural" juices, and all the foods filled with chemical flavorings, extenders, binders, and hybrid gluten that are "terrorizing" and destroying the intestinal tract and initiating chronic inflammation?

As children grow older, graduate from school, start a family or a business, the stress can be tremendous, perhaps even overwhelming. What does this do to all the stored toxins and inflammation that have been building up inside the intestinal tract during their developmental years? Even if they didn't have

ADHD, could this stress contribute to the onset of food sensitivities, allergies, rashes, celiac disease, fibromyalgia, etc.?

What happens when the body is overloaded with chemicals that have been accumulating for years, causing inflammation and dysfunction of body systems on such a gradual level that you don't even realize you are in trouble? How do you know if you are a slow ticking time bomb just waiting for the right element to trigger the explosion, and that trigger could just be simple stress? How easy would it be to change your diet and do things differently to change the outcome?

So, who is to blame for all this misery and degeneration? That is a tough question, because it is a soup mix of many generations of scientists, manufacturers, growers, producers, governments, retailers, and millions of consumers.

And what does the explosion bring? Just look around at all the people who are sick with so many different physical and mental incapacities. The death rate is too high in younger people with uncured diseases and undiagnosed misery. Change your diet now. Do everything you can to cleanse your body and teach your children how to eat better and live longer with good health and keen minds.

This year, 2014, the big food conglomerates are trying to stop GMO labeling. We must speak out and fight for the right to know what is in our food. If we don't get involved, then we have only ourselves to blame when things happen that we don't like or want.

People should use common sense in the choices they make about the food they eat. So much information is available to us that we can use the Internet to do our own research. Don't just accept what someone else says. Find the truth, be independent, and think for yourself. Set an example by what you do and say so that you can help others.

Without question, einkorn is the staff of life for our modern world. We have come full circle and now it is our responsibility to educate and teach our agricultural people the value of einkorn and encourage them to stop the hybridization of our grains and in turn stop the sickness that comes from eating them.

What is the answer? The answer can be very short or very long and complicated. The short answer is that we, the people, need to get involved and take responsibility for what is happening. We must become informed and share this information with those who are not informed, so we can grow in numbers and have a BIG voice when we speak out for our rights—our rights of life, liberty, and the pursuit of happiness.

The long way is the way to recovery if we don't take action now. It could be a long journey of pain and misery when we finally decide to change the path we are going down, a path that could end in disaster and eventually death, all because we just sat back and did nothing.

Yes, it's up to us. Do we want to know the truth, or will we suffer the consequences?

Yes, we want to know the truth, so let's take a stand and join with those who are like-minded to change the direction our world is going. Let's not wonder what is happening but be part of making things happen.

ENDNOTES

1   Klapp E, RD, BS. http://www.thediabetesclub.com/wp-content/plugins/downloads-manager/upload/Glycemic%20index%20food%20list.pdf.
2   http://www.huffingtonpost.com/dr-mark-hyman/wheat-gluten_b_1274872.html.